Caution: While reading Honey,  *you may guffaw yourself right into a v.) I'm telling you, this lady knov by name—and I recognize every een there—and am still doing that! True girl talk for the estrogen-deprived among us. Hooray, we are not alone!*

—Patsy Clairmont, Women of Faith Speaker;
Author, *Mending Your Heart in a Broken World*

I am one of those women Caron talks about in Honey, They Shrunk My Hormones—*too young to feel this old and in denial about the realities of midlife, while knowing it is inevitable. After all, my girlfriends are complaining of being hot and hostile. Yet, at forty-four, I am blessed by no physical signs of the pending doom. Through Caron's light touch and inclusive research, I now have an understanding of what is before me, I know that there are better ways to handle it than denial, and I see that there are perks amidst the pain—even rewards for living through it. I would never have read a medically oriented tome until I was in a state of crisis. Through this book I am both equipped and entertained.*

—Marita Littauer, President, CLASServices, Inc; Speaker;
Author of *You've Got What It Takes* and *Love Extravagantly*

Honey, They Shrunk My Hormones *is a laughter-filled journey into "middle age." We may not like it when our eyes start drooping, our shoulders start stooping, and our fat cells start grouping, but as Caron reminds us, getting older is definitely something to celebrate!*

So go on, get out the oxygen, take a deep breath, and blow out those birthday candles. Life is grand!

—Martha Bolton, Comedy Writer; Author of more than
fifty books, including *Didn't My Skin Used to Fit?*
and *The "Official" Hugs Book*

It has been said that we read books so we will not feel alone. Rarely has any book served that purpose so powerfully for women navigating the scary season of menopause. With her Christian perspective, refreshing honesty, and terrific sense of humor, Caron Loveless tackles even the most taboo topics of a woman's midlife journey. Pour yourself a cup of tea and dig into this treasure when the fears, discomforts, and anxieties of menopause threaten to overwhelm you.

—Nancy Beach, Teaching Pastor and Programming Director,
Willow Creek Community Church, South Barrington, Illinois

While I'm still on the other side of midlife, I'm glad to know that when I get there, I won't have to walk through that stage of life alone. In Honey, They Shrunk My Hormones, *Caron Loveless gives honest, vulnerable, and sometimes gut-wrenching glimpses into that season beyond youth. She shares with grace her experiences, fears, and surprise blessings that come with aging. Whether you're called a "ma'am," or you're still a "miss," you won't want to miss this girlfriend's guide to—gasp!—growing older.*

—Ginger Kolbaba, Managing Editor,
Marriage Partnership magazine

Honey, They Shrunk My Hormones

About the Author

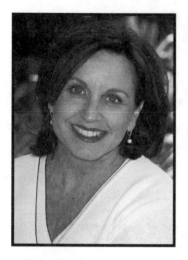

Caron Loveless is the creative director at Discovery Church in Orlando, Florida, where she and her husband, Senior Pastor David Loveless, have ministered together for eighteen of their twenty-seven years of marriage. They are the parents of three incredible sons and one beautiful daughter-in-love (who has just blessed them with their first grandchild).

When she is not keeping Hero off the kitchen counter, Caron is reading about writing, thinking about working out, or speaking in a church or conference somewhere in the uttermost parts of the United States or Canada. She has authored or coauthored nine other books, including *The Words That Inspired the Dreams* and the best-selling *Hugs from Heaven: Embraced by the Savior*. She has written articles for *Today's Christian Woman, Pastor's Family,* and other magazines, is a frequent guest on radio and television, and is a graduate of C.L.A.S.S. (Christian Leaders, Authors, and Speakers Seminar).

For information on how you can invite Caron to speak to your group or to tell your own midlife story, contact Caron at her Web site, www.caronloveless.com. Or write to her at: Discovery Church, 4400 S. Orange Avenue, Orlando, Florida, 32806. (www.discoverychurch.org)

Honey, They Shrunk My Hormones

Humor and Insight from the Trenches of Midlife

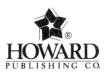

HOWARD
PUBLISHING CO.

Caron Chandler Loveless

Our purpose at Howard Publishing is to:

- *Increase faith* in the hearts of growing Christians
- *Inspire holiness* in the lives of believers
- *Instill hope* in the hearts of struggling people everywhere

Because He's coming again!

Honey, They Shrunk My Hormones © 2003 by Caron Chandler Loveless
All rights reserved. Printed in the United States of America
Published by Howard Publishing Co., Inc.
3117 North 7th Street, West Monroe, LA 71291-2227

03 04 05 06 07 08 09 10 11 12   10 9 8 7 6 5 4 3 2 1

Edited by Michele Buckingham
Cover design by Diane Whisner
Interior design by Stephanie Denney

Library of Congress Cataloging-in-Publication Data

Loveless, Carone, 1955-
    Honey, they shrunk my hormones! : humor and insight from the trenches of
midlife / Caron Chandler Loveless.
        p. cm.
    Includes bibliographical references.
    ISBN 1-58229-289-2
    1. Middle aged women. 2. Middle age. 3. Middle age—Humor. 4. Menopause.
5. Aging—Religious aspects—Christianity. I. Title.

HQ1059.4L67 2003
305.244—dc21

                                                                                              2002192183

Scripture quotations are taken from the HOLY BIBLE, NEW INTERNATIONAL VERSION®. Copyright © 1973, 1978, 1984 by International Bible Society. Used by permission of Zondervan Publishing House. All rights reserved.

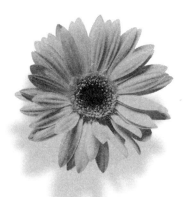

For
Lauren and Leslie,
who, rumor has it, used to get out of bed at night
and whisper through the wall outlets,
and who, even at *this late hour,* still let me be the big sister.

In loving memory of our mom,
Peggy Jo Chandler,

and for you,
my lady-boomer friend.

Just because everything is different,
doesn't mean anything has changed.
—Irene Peter

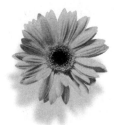

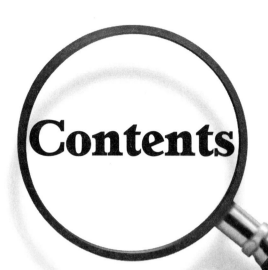

Contents

Part 3: Midlife Relationships: Holding On, Letting Go

Part 4: I Will Survive and Thrive

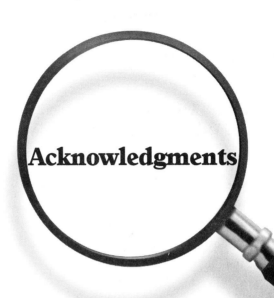

Acknowledgments

Writers are, for the most part, feeble, sensitive souls who need a good bit of prodding and propping to get their work done. At least that's the way it is with this writer. Knowing this fact, God assembled a small but effective army to nudge me toward the finish line.

Grateful thanks to my editors and friends, Philis and Denny Boultinghouse, for your ever-faithful encouragement and direction, and to the entire staff at Howard Publishing for giving me a place to share my heart. And to my new best friend and five-star editor, Michele Buckingham: *Mucho grande* kudos for taking the wad of flesh that was this book and adding the bones that make it stand up. You made a process that could feel like a root canal (minus the Novocaine) seem something akin to a pleasant dip in the sea.

Huge thanks to these dear friends and fellow authors: Christine Bolley, Martha Bolton, Patsy Clairmont, Suzie Duke,

Kristy Dykes, Deb Haggerty, Kathy Herman, Ginger Kolbaba, Marita Littauer, Janet Holm McHenry, Lindsey O'Connor, Pamela Smith, R.D., and LeAnn Weiss. Each of you stole precious time from your own projects to lend input and enthusiasm to mine; there is no greater gift.

Thanks also to Erica Smith. Your sweet willingness to read and edit blessed me so much.

Megathanks to the Discovery Church focus group girls: Diane Boles, Annette Botti, Lori Ann Buckley, Shirley Catella, June Chamberlin, Ginny Deloach, Joni Hansen, Mimi Jove, Patty Kalber, Suzan Lamp, Mary Lou Moss, Vivienne Moore, Corrie Moore, Cathy O'Neal, Robin Ragsdale, Cynthia Rollins, Pat Romo, Leslie Robinson, Julie Schuler, Suzanne Swyers, Sue Swain, and Lauren Walloch. Your humor and honesty bring spice to this book. Your hunger for Christ inspires me.

Thank you, my good friend and assistant, Leslie Aziz, for your beautiful chapter on midlife maternity and to Dale Hanson Bourke for the phrase used often in this book, the God Who Never Changes.

Grateful thanks to Lynn and Kent Shoemaker for your many instances of over-the-top generosity to my family and me during the writing of this book.

To my long-cherished friends and fellow ministers, Suzie Anfuso, Nancy Beach, Debbie Lord, and Martha Whitten: thank you. You will only know in heaven how much your friendship, your example of lives spent for Christ, and your *being there* have kept me in the race.

Special thanks, too, to these precious women who so willingly shared their midlives with me: Carrie Collins, Joann Smith, Renee Keller, Jackie Madsen, Susan Suttles, Lisa Lujan,

Anne Loewen, Kathy Johnston, Trish Smith and Susan, Wanda, Tante, Karen, and Grace from Park Avenue Baptist Church in Titusville, Florida.

A big thank-you to my creative planning team at Discovery Church: Leslie Aziz, Rocky Barra, Bernard Deloach, Darian Jaynes, Jay Mander, and Robin Ragsdale, who covered my bases and theirs, too—with no complaints—so I could finish this book.

To our sons, Joshua, Jonathan, and Joseph, and our daughter-in-love, Rebecca, my most precious, significant work in this world and God's hope for the next generation: Thank you for letting me tell our stories, checking on me throughout the process, smiling at all the right parts, explaining computer stuff so even I could understand it, and bringing me off-limits hamburgers. What a team. What a joy. It's been quite a ride. When you reach midlife, all of this nonsense will make sense.

Thank you, thank you, thank you to David, my handsome, patient prince, God's perfect gift to me, for cheering louder and longer than everyone else combined; for being extravagant with praise and stingy with criticism. Thank you for all the ways you grow your love for this midlife lady, who is not the same girl you married (but hopefully, in most ways, better). Boy, do I love you.

And thank you, Jesus—especially for the promise I cling to every day now: that you are the same yesterday, today, and forever.

PART 1

Midlife Is Real, and Real Women Go There

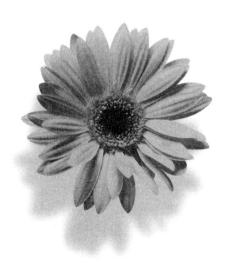

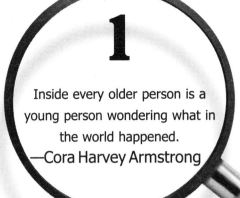

Inside every older person is a young person wondering what in the world happened.
—Cora Harvey Armstrong

Pardon Me, but Your Midlife Is Showing

Like most girls growing up, I had heard tales—myths—about a journey to the advanced State of Womanhood somewhere near a place called Mount Menopause. I knew some brave, ancient women who had ventured there. But what did they have to do with me? Those women were saggy and slow and bought shoes that were kind to their feet. I was young and thin (but a good eater) and could lay by the pool day after day—even at high noon—with nary a dab of sunscreen.

Then one husband, three children, and four pant sizes later, the wind shifted. A cold breeze blew in from the north, and with it came something like the sound of my first Timex watch.

For a while I couldn't place it, but then I knew: It was the tick-tick-tocking of a flesh-focused clock that the God Who Never Changes found necessary to install in me and you and every woman of every tribe and tongue, rich or poor, in sickness and in health (no thanks to Eve). Each year the clock got louder and louder, until its deafening sound woke me up most nights in a panicked sweat.

Then the ticking stopped. And there it was in the distance, no mistake: the first glimpse of that mythical Mount Menopause, spandexed across the horizon, big as my life.

With this revelation came the sudden urge for a fresh perspective. I knew I'd need wisdom beyond my current grasp if I hoped to scale the slippery slopes that loomed in front of me. So I took to scouring books and magazines, asking questions, and jotting down observations—until, finally, this book was born.

I don't know how close to the mountain you are, but trust me. Even if the evidence seems weak at the moment, before you can say, "You couldn't pay me to wear glasses," you will be hurled headlong into a maze of midlife odysseys that the God Who Never Changes allows in our lives in order to launch us (I believe) into an even higher altitude of feminine effectiveness.

Some days it feels like the end of the world, but it's not that at all. It's just the end of the world as we have known it. And as dreadful as that sounds, there are any number of upsides to one world slowing down and a new one cranking up, which we will explore in the pages ahead.

What's in It for You?

Perhaps you picked up this book because someone you care about is approaching midlife, and you think she could use a little boost. Okay, we can work with that.

Or maybe you are one of those women whose mother, wonderful as she was in so many ways, accidentally failed to mention the severity of certain anxiety-producing, heat-generating, life-altering experiences you are encountering right about now—and this omission has created a gnawing curiosity to find out what else she forgot to tell you. Or perhaps you've grown more than slightly annoyed with the uncertainty and inconvenience of this new life "season," and you wish someone would come along and help you sort some things out.

If these or other weird, uninvited feelings have begun pestering you, then, sister—honey, come on down!

If you are still clinging to the mid-to-upper thirties or lower forties, *Honey, They Shrunk My Hormones* can be your guidebook, chock-full of eyewitness, in-depth, gut-honest reporting intended to prove beyond reasonable doubt that, indeed, midlife is real, and real women go there.

If you are heavily invested in your forties—or beyond—you might consider the volume you hold as a lifeline. Its most significant benefit will be the comfort and cheer you'll get from knowing that a woman much like you is surviving and learning to thrive through this often uncertain "phase"—even if her kids do think they can make it without her, and her mind has put up a vacancy sign, and she does have some "back fat" (plus a mean set of bunions), and she might as well not own the World's Most Comfortable Bed for as little sleep as she gets these days.

Honey, They Shrunk My Hormones is about way more than estrogen, progesterone, and night sweats (though we do give these topics an honorable mention). Consider this book a virtual micropedia of the joys and afflictions that often accompany women in "second adulthood." In its pages:

- You will be taken for a wild, *Consumer Report*-like ride with a frightened first-time mammogram-ee.

- Certain strange, new developments will be openly confessed.

- You'll meet the cute, bouncy girls at my local health club.

- I will attempt to prove that if the Eternal God and Father of our Lord Jesus Christ doesn't have an earth age, then we probably don't either.

- We'll consider the immense value of a little "good grief."

- We'll also kick around how it feels to dismantle the family you've spent twenty-some years constructing; the importance of a good pair of tweezers; what to do the first time someone calls you the G-word; and 122 semisignificant things we should probably know by now. And that just gets us started.

It's Not Just Me

Just so you know, in order to keep this book from solely being skewed from my perspective, I sent a carload of midlife questionnaires to strangers, family, and friends in places like Maui, Hawaii; Greensboro, North Carolina; Chicago, Illinois; British Columbia, Canada; and Titusville, Florida. You can read excerpts of some of the frank and funny responses I received from them in the sections called "In the Chat Room."

Most of the women in the chat rooms are married with children. Some are single, divorced, or widowed. Some are in second marriages. A few have babies and preschoolers, some have kids in elementary, but most have preteens or older. They are nurses, office assistants, teachers, sales managers, estheticians, small-business owners, full-time moms and homemakers, and women in full-time ministry. The statements are their own, with minor editing. A few names were changed by request.

In addition to sending out questionnaires, I gathered two focus groups of midlife-ish women in my home for two nights of midlife girl talk. Chapter 3 is a composite of those meetings.

And then, since I did not have children later in life, I asked my good friend, Leslie Aziz, to share her musings on the experience of midlife maternity. Those are found in chapter 15.

All together, what you hold in your hands is a gift to you and your friends: a collection of lip-grinning, heart-nudging, truth-telling talks about our thrill ride as midlifing women. It is an eclectic collage of some of the issues we all face at this curious stage in our lives. Ultimately, it is an unveiling of many of the things God wants us to learn and to become—taught in the furnace of the most significant, most stretching, and most glorious growing up he has ever asked us to do.

I hope you laugh. A page or two might make you cry. Mostly, I hope you're encouraged to find that you're taking this trip in good company.

But I trust in you, O LORD; I say, "You are my God." My times are in your hands. (Ps. 31:14-15)

⟡ ⟡ In the Chat Room

Anne, 48: *"Midlife seemed to come too soon. I wish I had enjoyed my twenties and thirties more, when I didn't have hot flashes, gray hair, kids leaving home, low sex drive, parents to care for, and wrinkles."*

Joann, 59: *"When you're older, people think you're wise; they don't expect vitality and bubbly bouncing around. If you bubble and bounce, they're amazed. You don't have to worry about being pretty all the time, which is freeing."*

Mary Lou, 51: *"I work with younger people, and that keeps me young. I don't think they view me as much different from them."*

Martha, 49: *"In my younger years I depended on my appearance to gain favor, so I feel I have to get over that shallow way of relating now."*

Jackie, 46: *"It always surprises me when others don't view me as a young person—like the time I was riding the hospital elevator up to the maternity floor where I work, and a lady asked if I was a new grandmother!"*

Annette, 46: *"I still feel as if I'm in my twenties."*

Ginny, 42: *"I see my daughter doing cartwheels and splits and can't believe I can't do them anymore."*

June, 59: *"I try not to focus on my physical self as much; I try to look past the exterior. In fact, I find myself much happier when I keep the focus off myself and put it more on others. Self-image is just not that important to me anymore. But when I look in the mirror, the person I see on the outside is not who I feel like on the inside."*

Cathy, 42: *"The fact that I look older doesn't bother me, because I know who I am in Christ. I'm a result of all the experiences God has allowed in my life."*

2

I can be changed by what
happens to me,
but I am not reduced by it.
—Maya Angelou

Has Anyone Seen
My Hormones?

If there is one word most associated with middle-aged women,
it's *hormones*. Everywhere you turn, it seems, our hormones are
on display. They're in the news, in commercials, on billboards, at
the doctor's office, in magazines, on talk radio—(not to mention
certain catchy book titles). Yet despite all the day-in and day-out
publicity given to our fickle, fluctuating endocrine glands, there
are still a number of mysteries that we need to solve.

For example, why, when we're in the prime of our lives, is it
suddenly necessary for our female hormones (which were doing
just fine) to shrink, and for other hormones (dare I say, *male*-type
hormones) to surge? Since you've probably been puzzled by the

same question, I'd like to share with you my own theory on this highly disturbing subject.

To be perfectly ethical, let me say up front that the scientific community has yet to recognize this theory. But anyone who has ever seen the movie *Back to the Future 2* knows that while scientists are, by and large, brilliant and can, even without the aid of a calculator, predict with pinpoint accuracy how long it will take a Siamese cat traveling at mach three on the back of a killer whale to orbit Pluto and return to Earth, they are still light-years away from unraveling *all* of life's unsolved mysteries—particularly the ones having to do with the female anatomy.

In other words, on this subject, my guess is as good as theirs. And I think it's within the realm of possibility that at the point of conception, we girls are given a microscopic squirt of male hormones that lie perfectly dormant in our bodies for, oddly enough, about the same time it took the children of Israel to find the Promised Land. Meanwhile, our counterparts (the boys) are blessed at conception with a generous, God-given glut of male hormones that pretty much have a field day for decades riding broncos, racing monster trucks, and bursting water balloons on poor, unsuspecting motorists.

Then one day out of sheer exhaustion (check this out: also around age forty), the man's hormones begin to fizzle out. How do we know this? A sure sign that a man is minus some male hormones is when you see him slumped on the couch watching cooking shows and showing zero interest in stalking his wife around the house like he used to.

Now comes what I call the "hormonal fruit basket turnover." In an effort to help us make good (to the very end) on his command to "be fruitful and increase" (Gen. 1:28), at this crucial point God arranges for the wife's secret stash of male hormones to briefly—but briskly—kick in. Suddenly, out of the blue, *she* becomes loud, aggressive, and even runs around the house stalking her husband. (And sometimes he lets her catch him!)

So there you have it: a perfectly reasonable explanation for the confusing, schizoid behavior of midlife females—and for all those cute little late-in-life "surprises" we see born to some stunned midlife couples.

Entering Midlife U

I don't know why more people haven't picked up on this theory. I suppose it *is* hard to stay current with all the latest biological breakthroughs in women's health these days. But no one ever told us that in order to survive this season of life, we would have to become proficient in pharmacology, psychology, biology, endocrinology, physiology, cardiology, oncology, dermatology, gynecology, ophthalmology, theology, proctology, cosmetology, podiatry, and naturopathy, not to mention reading. (Think of all that fine print on your vitamin labels.) Burdened with a class load like this, no wonder we sometimes get cranky.

Of course the men at my house claim to have my hormone fluctuations down to a science. They say that even from a distance, they can spot my hormonal juices percolating. According to these guys, at the slightest rise in my vocal pitch, a sophisticated audio detection device gets triggered in their brains, alerting them to head for the garage and hand out the riot gear. You'd think this would offend me or hurt my feelings, but it doesn't. I am very much aware that these guys are men, and at certain times *their* hormones get cooped up and need a little workout. So you see, all things do work together for good.

Fortunately, God made the reorganization of a woman's

hormonal structure a *gradual* process. Which we appreciate, because if we went through the change overnight, upon entering the menopausal atmosphere we would instantly incinerate —since, some experts say that a single hot flash is capable of raising a woman's temperature seven or eight degrees in mere seconds. Special consideration—and lots of room—must be given to those women who go through the change overnight by way of a hysterectomy. I won't get into this procedure here except to note, in passing, the curious correlation between it and the word *hysteria*.

Decisions, Decisions, Decisions

These days women are asked to make a lot of crucial decisions about their bodies. Again, we try; but it takes a genius to figure out which piece of advice has our name on it. Should we take hormone replacement therapy (HRT) and take our chances with an increased risk of breast cancer, or should we forgo HRT and die someday from the complications of osteoporosis? Are we or are we not helped by HRT in the heart disease department? Will we gain more weight on HRT as some report, or lose, as others claim?

Experts say we should go all-natural. Other experts say we should do HRT for its long-term benefits. Wise women take HRT. Other wise women do not. Always, it seems, a new study comes out to sway us from believing the last one that proclaimed it was the definitive word on the subject.

Experts tell us that estrogen is involved in at least *three hundred* bodily processes. And when it dips below levels the body has come to expect for thirty years, no wonder chaos ensues. Apparently, everything from the brain to the hypothalamus gets confused, and with that goes the regulation of our sleep, temperature, appetite, libido, periods, and general sense of well-being.

The fact is, each of us possesses our own unique blend of flustered internal circuitry. Gail Sheehy, in her book *New Passages: Mapping Your Life Across Time*, writes: "Menopause is as individual as a thumbprint. No two women experience it alike."[1] That means we can't simply do what our friends are doing; we may not have the same symptoms or feel them with equal intensity. Sheehy also writes that some 20 percent of us will breeze through menopause with nary a scratch, while the other 80 percent will have to cope with multiple combinations of twenty different menopausal (and premenopausal) symptoms.[2] As a result, narrowing down the best options *for us* may take months, even years. It's enough to make a girl pull her hair out—if she has some to spare.

Prescription for Progress

When it comes to these kinds of choices, I've decided to live by three phrases: *read it, weigh it,* then *test it.*

Reading is easy. We certainly don't lack for information on this subject. A plethora of books, medical pamphlets, and Web sites dedicated to women's health are available to help you make informed decisions about your body. I have to admit that for a long time my problem was not finding the data; it was carving out time to do the research. I have several good books on the shelf. I just didn't stop long enough to study them early on. As a result I endured a number of uncomfortable symptoms longer than I probably needed to.

Weighing the information is more of a challenge. I've found that it helps if you list your symptoms then compare both the natural and pharmaceutical options for relieving them. An important person in this process is your doctor. Make sure you have an OB/GYN you can trust—someone you're confident will give you the best medical counsel based on your one-of-a-kind needs. If you don't have a doctor you can talk to, make the effort to find a woman's hormonal health specialist in your area.

Don't just talk to medical people, however. Ask God for his mind on this matter. After all, he's the one who created you and your hormones. I learned this one the hard way. Even though I knew better; even though I often quoted, "If any of you lacks wisdom, he should ask God, who gives generously" (James 1:5); even though I understood that all decisions are ultimately spiritual decisions—still it wasn't until I reached a boiling point that I realized I hadn't consulted the Holy Spirit about my changing hormonal situation.

If you're married, why not ask your husband to pray with you? And while you're at it, share crucial information with him. Invite his input. Then go the way that brings you the most peace.

Testing the results of different options can take months or more. To be honest, I've found the waiting part hard. I want to see immediate change—in a week or so, tops—and if that doesn't happen, I'm tempted to throw out that option and try another. At this point I've tried three or four remedies, and I'm not quite satisfied that I have the right mix for me yet.

But, hey, I've been thinking. If I *have* to go through the rigors of gone-haywire, fever-spiking hormonal changes, then the fact that I live in Florida is an advantage. When I go out, I can still mix with the locals without fear of getting caught in the middle of a hot flash. Down here, like it or not, sweat just comes with the territory.

You teach me wisdom in the inmost place. (Ps. 51:6)

⚉ ⚉ In the Chat Room

Karen, 65: *"I take Premarin. It's supposedly good for the bones and heart and for eliminating hot flashes. At first I just went along with the doctor and took it. Then I heard it was made from pregnant horse urine, and I stopped taking it. The hot flashes returned, so I said, 'Oh, well,' and started taking it again. It's okay."*

Lisa, 47: *"My bones and muscles remind me that I'm not young anymore. Lack of sleep, poor diet, being on the go—I can't get away with these things like I used to. My body puts me in my place. It just refuses to cooperate."*

Anne, 48: *"I take estrogen and progesterone. I never thought I would. But the hot flashes are completely gone now! I hated them."*

June, 59: *"I had a hysterectomy, so I've taken Premarin for the past eighteen years. My doctor said it would keep me from 'drying up like an old prune.' I don't know. I guess I would have been worse without it."*

Patricia, 49: *"I take FemHRT. I resisted at first, but I finally surrendered a year ago and consented to take it every other day. It makes the hot flashes milder, and it helps with the mood swings, so I guess it's worth it."*

Shelley, 51: *"I didn't want to take HRT, so a doctor told me to take herbs instead. They help me with vaginal dryness and depression, and my hot flashes are totally gone. I haven't heard a lot of good stuff about HRT."*

Joann, 59: *"I take estrogen. I feel much better—definitely positive results. Before my hormone replacement kicked in, my family sometimes just stared at me, wide-eyed over something outrageous I'd said."*

Martha, 49: *"I was having a tendency toward mood swings and being introverted and somewhat depressed. My husband noticed my desire to stay home more, to not have to go out and get up for other people's expectations. I'm generally more outgoing. Hormones have helped with this considerably."*

Susan, 49: *"I don't take hormones, just vitamins and minerals."*

Resources to Help Beat the Heat

Web sites

www.pamsmith.com—Pamela Smith, R.D., is a nationally known Christian nutritionist. Her excellent Web site features many books, tapes, and other materials designed to help women take charge of the change (and other aspects of their health and well-being).

www.womens-health.com—This is a fascinating interactive Web site designed to help you assess your health through a series of diagnostic questions. It also provides a wide range of informative articles and research on issues most relevant to you.

www.midlife-passages.com—This site offers research and information directly related to midlife for both men and women.

Books

Take Charge of the Change by Pamela Smith, R.D.

What Your Doctor May Not Tell You about Premenopause by John R. Lee, M.D.

The Wisdom of Menopause by Christiane Northrup, M.D.

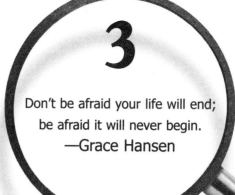

3

Don't be afraid your life will end;
be afraid it will never begin.
—Grace Hansen

Wombs to Go

I missed another period this month. This is the second time I've done it but the first time I've stopped to contemplate how I feel about it.

I know. This is supposed to be happening. I'm nearing the Big Kahuna. But I've been so distracted by the night sweats, acne, and general weirdness that comes with perimenopause that I haven't taken the time to think about how I will feel when my ovaries finally go out of business.

Curious George

"George" came for his inaugural visit when I was ten years old. Like underworld spies, Pamela Bender and I found it necessary to use a code name for our new monthly guest. "Oh, George came today," we'd say. Or, "Sorry, I can't go swimming. You know, George is here."

George was a curious phenomenon, and, according to the film they showed us in Girl Scouts, we should view it as sort of a red badge of womanhood. On the day this film was shown, our mothers were invited to join us under the guise of a mother-daughter tea. With great attention to detail, "menstruation" was unveiled, and I, the queen of modesty, sat cringing at the thought of my stepmother listening in the back of the room. "Menstruation" was a concept few of us girls could grasp or even pronounce, and we gawked in puzzlement at a woman's inner workings, which, to me, looked a lot like a steer head skeleton—the kind you might see hanging on a fence post out West. Looking back, I'd say the film was probably a good idea, since my mom never turned out to be a wealth of information on the more intimate matters.

My friend George (in those days he was our friend) actually arrived with a fright on January 12, first thing in the morning. I remember because it was my sister's birthday. While taking my turn in the bathroom, I was horrified to find a large crimson stain on my underwear. Because mom had been so hush-hush about the matter and because the little bits of information I had garnered over the years had seemed so mysterious—I stole off, stain and all, to school drenched in the shame of a first-time criminal.

In P.E. I whispered to Pamela Bender that I was in real trouble, that I had found some blood and didn't know what to do.

"Oh my gosh!" Pam whispered back. "We should tell the teacher."

"No, we can't do that. She'd tell my mom."

"Well, you're going to have to tell her sooner or later."

"I will…later."

The thought of that inevitable "later" filled me with such dread that I was sick with fear through the rest of the day and evening.

We had a party for my sister that night, and when the birthday guests were gone, I knew I couldn't stall any longer. Leading Mom to my room, I guiltily opened my pajama drawer, pulled out the incriminating evidence, and waited for the ax to fall.

I was floored by her response. "Well," she said, half grinning, "I guess you're becoming a woman."

And with that I was marched swiftly into the bathroom to receive my first and only instruction in the feminine art of napkin wearing, which involved (you might remember) the hooking of the gauzy ends of a Kotex pad through the metal clasps of a weird, elastic, beltlike contraption.

That night, protected to the hilt, I lay smiling in the dark, feeling the kind of immense relief you get when you wake up from a bad dream and find that you did not kill your teacher after all. *I haven't done anything wrong,* I thought. *I'm just becoming a woman.*

So What *Is* a Woman?

It is now thirty-seven years and four-hundred-forty-four cycles later (take away fifty or so for pregnancies, nursing, and miscarriages), and I'm wondering if a part of what makes me regret the dawning of menopause is a kind of subconscious thinking that goes: *If the onset of menstruation makes a woman out of me, does the ceasing of it make me not one?*

Of course, no one would actually come out and say, "You are no longer a woman after menopause," but the fact that for decades we've had the period-womanhood connection drilled into our heads must at least *contribute* to the confusion we feel as our periods start to decrease.

Letty Cottin Pogrebin, in her book *Getting Over Getting Older*, says:

> I expect to live more than one-third of my life post-menopausally, and while I'm sure I will be a somewhat dif-ferent person in the next thirty years, it will not be because I stopped having periods. I see no reason to give this physio-logical development any more notice than I gave puberty once it had accomplished its purpose....I didn't think of myself as "postpubescent," and at this point, I'm not willing to be defined as "postmenopausal" when a dozen other iden-tities are more descriptive.[1]

When I first read that passage, I couldn't help but wonder: *How will I define myself when there are no more calendars to watch, tampons to buy, or cramps to endure?*

Someone suggested that I should look at my failing womb like a piece of equipment that has outlived its usefulness. But when my blender breaks down or my purse wears out, I buy a new one. Obviously there are no replacement wombs (at least not this year). And being on the verge of forty-seven years old, I don't think I would want one anyway.

Through the years my period has brought me everything from elation to irritation to inconvenience and despair. When it is gone, I will not miss the swelling, the edginess, or the rav-enous appetite that came with it. I will not miss having to say to someone I've hurt, "Sorry, you'll have to be patient with me. I guess it's that time of the month."

So what is the problem?

Midcourse Correction

When it comes down to it, I think what bothers me most about the approach of menopause is the sobering fact that a part of me is, let's face it…dying. Menopause will be one more reminder that all things in this world will—*must*—pass away. And yet it is also a reminder that Christ's claim on my life transcends death, since he calls me to live and serve with him every day at that higher place where nothing ever dies.

In the past a "mortal womb" announced to the world, "She's rounding the bend, folks. She's heading into the home stretch. Her fruitful days are over." But this is a new day. We are the first generation to benefit not only from an emphasis on nutrition and exercise but also from an avalanche of scientific breakthroughs. We have the potential to remain vibrant and healthy well into old age. And that's great, since the biblical evidence is clear that our God Who Never Changes is adamant about his people bearing much fruit at every stage of their lives.

Sooner rather than later, it will be obvious that one very female part of our bodies is closing up shop. But let's remind each other that this is just one storefront in the whole thriving metropolis that is our life. When it happens, we can let it be a sign, a commissioning, a call to fling wide the door of our hearts to a new, fertile place of influence and productiveness. Instead of thinking, *Sorry, old girl. Time's up*, let's tell ourselves and one another, "Okay, so our energies are needed elsewhere now. It's time to get a move on. Let's see where God wants us next."

⊡ ⊡ In the Chat Room

Jackie, 46: *"I take birth control pills to regulate my periods, which could be considered a form of hormone replacement. I've taken them since I was thirty and plan to continue until menopause. They help manage my PMS and perimenopausal symptoms, which have worsened as I've gotten older."*

Martha, 49: *"After I stopped having periods, I fought the idea of taking hormones for a year because of horror stories. In that time, my skin dried up, my bones weakened, and I became introverted and weird. I'm so glad I started taking hormone replacements because I feel back to the real me, and my skin looks better. My husband has noticed the difference."*

Ginny, 42: *"I'm really tired of having periods!"*

Lu Anne, 37: *"My husband jokes that we have one good week a month— because one week I'm ovulating, one week I have PMS, and one week I have my period."*

Pat, 49: *"Ironically, as my daughter [from a previous marriage] is moving into puberty and nearing the onset of menstruation, that chapter is ending for me. This is sad because my husband and I have only been married four years and would have loved to have had a child together."*

But I am like an olive tree flourishing in the house of God;
I trust in God's unfailing love for ever and ever. (Ps. 52:8)

Becoming a Farsighted Female

Read the following scriptures in light of the many changes you are facing at this time in your life. Ask the Holy Spirit to give you eyes to see and a heart to embrace that next new place of fruitfulness that God is preparing for you.

1. "Therefore, since we are surrounded by such a great cloud of witnesses, let us throw off everything that hinders and the sin that so easily entangles, and let us run with perseverance the race marked out for us." (Heb. 12:1)

   Ask God: What things easily entangle me? What does the race that you have marked out *for me* look like?

2. "Therefore, I urge you, brothers, in view of God's mercy, to offer your bodies as living sacrifices, holy and pleasing to God—this is your spiritual act of worship." (Rom. 12:1)

   Ask God: How can I offer my body to you as a living, holy sacrifice? What would please you most?

3. "However, as it is written: 'No eye has seen, no ear has heard, no mind has conceived what God has prepared for those who love him'—but God has revealed it to us by his Spirit." (1 Cor. 2:9–10)

   Ask God: What things do you want me to know about the future that you have prepared for me? How can I love you more?

4. "Forget the former things; do not dwell on the past. See, I am doing a new thing! Now it springs up; do you not perceive it? I am making a way in the desert and streams in the wasteland." (Isa. 43:18–19)

Ask God: What former things am I still holding on to? What is the new thing you want to do with me?

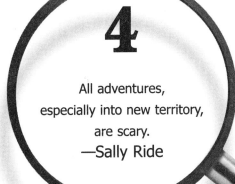

4

All adventures,
especially into new territory,
are scary.
—Sally Ride

If You Can't Stand the Heat, You're Not Alone

Giddy and chatty, they invade my house, a gumbo of heights, weights, and hair dyes.

"Where should I put my purse?" says one.

"Everyone needs a nametag," says another.

Some of these women are long-time friends. Others will leave here with new friends. Among us is a teacher, an administrator, a water-ski instructor, a nurse, a realtor, a full-time mom and homemaker, a stage manager, a sales manager, an X-ray technician, a church staff member, a medical assistant, and a small-business owner. It's a diverse group. What brings us together tonight? Our age.

This is a midlife focus group—a first for them and for me. None of us has talked about the challenges of our unique stage of life "officially," and we're anxious to see what will happen as the night progresses.

To get the women here, I have promised them exotic, no-cal delights; intimate talk on a subject we'd all rather avoid; considerable laughter; and a future copy of *Honey, They Shrunk My Hormones,* which (at the time of this meeting) is still in the larvae stage.

Juggling snacks and drink bottles, we circle up chairs and wriggle in on the sofa. On my lap is a yellow notepad filled with more questions than we will have time to answer. They think my plan is to glean all of their secrets and pass the stack on to you. But the truth is, I have asked them here to teach me.

"Did you bring your questionnaires?" I say.

Blank stares.

Then someone says, "We were supposed to bring those?"

"Oh, I forgot mine."

"Me too."

"The brain is the first thing to go."

"That's the truth!"

We go around the room and tell our names, ages, and, to warm things up, our favorite places to shop. The age part gets some guff, though. Some joke to duck the question. But one thing I'm firm on: no hedging. Soon we know that the youngest among us is thirty-seven; the oldest, fifty-nine.

Before we begin our discussion, I want to hear God's voice in the room, give him a chance to speak first. So I quiet everyone down, open my Bible, and read: "There is a time for everything (pause), and a season for every activity under heaven (long pause):

a time to be born and a time to die,

a time to plant and a time to uproot...

a time to tear down and a time to build,

a time to weep and a time to laugh...

a time to scatter stones and a time to gather them,

a time to embrace and a time to refrain...

a time to keep and a time to throw away...

a time to be silent and a time to speak...

The room is still. Some eyes go moist. Tonight these truths seem sobering. We hear the words and see a part of our lives floating past—or perhaps a part we dread facing drawing nearer. As a group we melt and merge.

I continue: "He has made everything beautiful in its time. He has also set eternity in the hearts of men; yet they cannot fathom what God has done from beginning to end" (Eccles. 3:1–7, 11). The words never seemed truer than now.

Then we grab hands, and I pray: "Oh, Lord, you are truly the God Who Never Changes. You're also the God of all seasons. We know that. We've seen that. You made us. You know our frames. Help us to see your purpose in this new and confusing stage in our lives. Help us to make some sense of it. Help us to trust you in it. And help us to make you proud."

We sit for a moment in silence. Then I dive in.

Why Didn't Someone Tell Us?

"Well, guys, just two rules," I say. "Number one, no subject is off limits. Say whatever you like. And number two, everyone has to share—no spectators. Okay?"

A few heads nod. Then I ask, "How many of you felt ready for midlife—you know, felt somewhat prepared?"

No one budges.

"Okay, how many did *not* feel prepared?"

Hands fly up, and with them, the chatter. *No one* felt clued in or ready. Many admit that they still don't.

"So what's going on?" I ask. "Why do you think this is? Why are we not prepared for this season?"

"I've been so busy working and running around with the kids," one pipes up. "I didn't even see it coming. It happened so out of the blue. Sounds silly, I know, but I always thought midlife was for older people, not someone young like me."

There's laughter, more chatter, a series of nods and nudges.

"My mother never talked about midlife," another says. "She never mentioned it or complained about symptoms, so I never thought anything of it. I guess, in her time, you just didn't talk about this sort of thing. Basically, I've been pretty ignorant."

Again, there's group consensus.

One by one the women put into words what I've been feeling: low on female instruction, blindsided as a whole. I had figured that, surely, I was a freak. I'm surprised to hear that these bright, educated women aren't on top of this thing, either.

In fact, a corporate sigh of relief fills the air as one, then another, then another admits how midlife has caught her off guard, how much she still doesn't know. Only two women say they have read books on the subject. Many confess that they've come to this meeting hoping to learn something new.

Midlife in a Nutshell

I ask them to describe midlife in one or two words, and here's what comes out: Hard. Unpredictable. Exciting. Irritating.

Illogical. Frustrating. High maintenance. Discombobulated. Full and tough. Hot and wet! Roller coaster. Happy and challenging. Confusing. Stretching. Scary. Full and empty. Better perspective. More wisdom. Freedom. Empty nest. Grace under fire. A glorious unexpected.

A *glorious unexpected*? This comment comes from one of the older women. I wonder if a pattern is forming along age lines.

"I almost didn't come tonight," the youngest says. "This whole subject depresses me."

"Honestly, I never thought I would be anything but young," another younger one admits. "I sure don't feel as if I'm 'midlife.'"

"Well, I'm having the time of my life," the oldest among us offers. "I have nothing to lose now. When I turned fifty-two— that was really tough. I thought I'd never make it through that year. But you girls just wait. It gets better! Really. You get to the point where all the fuss and work of always trying to look good for people just isn't important anymore. I'm closer to God now than ever. I have great purpose through the serving I do at church. Even though I'm widowed and live alone, I love my life. I wouldn't trade ages with any of you—*bodies*, maybe, but not ages."

No one speaks, but by the looks on their faces, I know what many of them are thinking: *What planet is this lady from?*

It occurs to me that the women in the group who have passed through menopause seem happier, more settled, more resilient than the rest of us. They have been through the fiery forties and have come out on the other side. I have read about postmenopausal zest, and some of these women have it. They have more focus about them and a spiritual depth and curiosity that is highly attractive—but that seems light-years from where I sit right now.

Learning from One Another

For the next two hours we take turns spilling our stories, our fears, and our confusions. We laugh, get teary-eyed, and commiserate. We're surprised to hear that there are others like us. Our most common traits are our unpreparedness for midlife, our stubborn refusal to get "old," and our silent mothers who never talked about their own experiences. Most of us have been so busy working or raising kids that we've never stopped to notice the new stage of life we're in. A kind of shell shock prevails.

All through the night I hear, "Yes!"

"That's right!"

"Me too!"

We seem like a herd of schoolgirls lost in the woods and in search of their teacher. But tonight these schoolgirls are teaching me a few things:

- We are greatly confused about midlife. But at least now we know that we aren't hallucinating, and we're not as alone as we thought. This gives us courage.

- We're bewildered at how fast life is speeding by. Can we really be at this point already?

- We all get depressed and weird and lash out and have irrational fears that we've never felt before. Sometimes we isolate ourselves and don't even realize we're doing it.

- We really don't like how we look, and we feel helpless to change it.

- We're frustrated about all the contradictions we hear about hormone replacement therapy. Some of us take hormones; most of us don't. All of us hope that we're making the best choices for us.

- We like our kids better now.

- We like ourselves better now. We're wiser, more experienced, and most days, more confident.

- Our marriages seem better, too, although we're not as interested in sex. And the gap created by children leaving home does create fallout in some relationships.

- We love the assurance laughter brings.

- We're glad we have good friends and a God Who Never Changes.

Clearly, this is not our mothers' midlife. But tonight we have gained a sense of sisterhood, a special kinship born for such a season as this. Everyone wants a repeat. We want to talk again and support each other. Some want to start a small group. Others would love a retreat.

One thing we definitely agree on: Simply being together helps. Gathering in one room, confronting our issues aloud, seeing ourselves in others—these things have a mystical way of easing our anxiety and making midlife seem doable. As the evening ends, we're more hopeful than ever that good things *do* exist on the other side of Mount Menopause.

If we can just hang on through the rocky parts.

☜ ☞ In the Chat Room

Shirlee, 51: *"When I look in the mirror, I think, 'Geesh! Nice looking neck!' But I don't hang on to stuff like I used to—like, 'If you want to fire me, fire me. Whatever.' Ego dies down. Life gets more poignant and streamlined."*

Jackie, 46: *"In some ways my self-image is better now. I'm more accepting of myself. But I am having trouble gaining perspective about all the physical changes. I've got thinning hair, sagging everything, age spots, wrinkles, thicker ankles, old-looking hands, and they all bother me!"*

Carrie, 44: *"I finally cut twelve inches off my hair. I care what my blood pressure is and whether or not my house will be paid off before I have to retire. I would still like to get married; there's hope. But I'd like to tie a knot into women who are not self-sufficient. Some women think they can't survive without a man."*

Suzie, 52: *"I'm more secure and stronger about my opinions now, which is an adjustment for my husband. It doesn't really matter what people think of me. I have a goal to age gracefully and be an example to younger women who fight the physical aspects of aging."*

June, 59: *"Widowed in midlife, overcoming all that goes with that, being suddenly alone, no prospects for the future, trying to care for two homes by myself—the responsibility was huge. I used to pray, 'Please, God, find me a man.' Now I pray, 'Thank you, God, for not bringing me a man!' I love being single."*

And our hope for you is firm, because we know that just as you share in our sufferings, so also you share in our comfort. (2 Cor. 1:7)

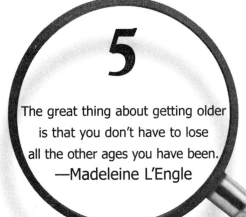

The great thing about getting older
is that you don't have to lose
all the other ages you have been.
—Madeleine L'Engle

Everybody's Doing the Birthday Bash

Women, especially maturing ones, are world renowned for singing the birthday blues. Every once in a while a guy might pipe in with a lament about his age; but for the most part, we girls have a monopoly on the market. It seems we just can't get past the numbers.

One woman with a stellar reputation for hiding her true age was pioneer cosmetic queen Elizabeth Arden, who once was quoted as saying, "I'm not interested in age. People who tell me their age are silly. You're only as old as you feel." But Ms. Arden was obsessed with aging. By the time she died, her age had been hidden so well that her obituary was off nearly ten years.

Is Age Ever Beautiful?

Why are we so ashamed of our age? Where does this attitude come from? We don't feel this way about the ages of other things.

Take trees, for instance. Where I live, people will go to ridiculous extremes to save a seventy-year-old oak tree from the lumber pile. They'll chain themselves to the trunk, daring developers to crank up their saws. Or take wine. In certain parts of the world, aged wine is practically sacred. We hear things like, "Fifty-six was a very good year, no?" "Ahhh, yes, my friend. But forty-seven, now *that* was the year, was it not?" With wine, age is everything.

We even build monuments to aged things. We charge admission to see prehistoric finger bowls worth more than the gross national product of Paraguay. Really old art gets round-the-clock security, keeping everyone under surveillance to ensure that some child's Cheeto-ed hand doesn't go for the pharaoh's Tupperware.

We hoard old things. It doesn't matter what they are, as long as they can be proven to be authentically old. As we speak, there is no doubt someone in Virginia or Tennessee who has a priceless assortment of Civil War toothpicks that she wouldn't part with if you paid her. And then there's the quirky world of antiques, where the operative word is *circa*. If you have something with a really old circa, folks will come from miles around to take their picture with it.

In these certain "acceptable areas," old is beautiful, valuable, honorable. So why don't we apply those same adjectives to ourselves? Why do we squirm when someone asks our age? Why do we leave the age line blank on questionnaires? Why are we relieved to learn that someone else is older than we are?

Is Youth Really Everything?

You could answer by saying that in today's appearance-driven economy, the movers and shakers who make all the decisions only value "pretty, young things." You could add that movies and advertisements are geared for Generation Next, and that makes the rest of us chopped liver. You could point to real-life incidents in which aging TV anchorwomen have been let go or repositioned to age gracefully just out of camera range. You could also admit that you have gotten a little attached to "feeling young" yourself—and who, in all honesty, would not prefer a sleek, late-model car to an oil-dripping, clunky old heap?

You could say all of that, and on many days I would be right there agreeing with you. But even if the whole earth worships at the temple of Youth, I can't help but wonder: Do you and I—and millions of other smart, seasoned, spiritual women like us—really have to be age-a-phobic?

Trying to trace my own thinking on the subject, I flipped through my journals looking for an entry I made on my fortieth birthday. Here's what I wrote:

April 2, 1995

It's almost as if this birthday were happening to someone else. I don't feel what I think forty is supposed to feel like. Yet it is my birthday, and I must somehow own it and receive this day for all it brings to me. Four decades of my life have now passed. Sometime I should give names to these decades and see what they would be called.

If I get to live long, I am already halfway. It's halftime. But I really don't want to come out of the locker room, for then I will be forced to finish the game, win or lose. Regardless of how I play, the clock will run toward the sound of the buzzer, of that I am sure. But today I'm afraid I will use up too much of the clock trying to decide which play to run or getting into position for a great score.

Today is my fortieth birthday! Forty is the dividing line of outward beauty. There aren't many over-forty supermodels. But perhaps forty is the onset of a more internal beauty that stays secure throughout the further seasons of body and soul. At least that is what I'm told and what I desperately wish to believe.

I cannot dwell too long today on where I have not gone and what I have not done, or the friends I have lost and the weight I have gained. For today is what it is: a mile marker, an imaginary remembrance of the day I was brought into this world to take part in it. A day for remembering that I started somewhere and I will finish somewhere else, and my whole life, such as it is, will be lived between those two defining posts.

Today is for saying to myself, "Yes, the day is getting on, but it's not too late to live within it fully."

I feel hopeful today—hopeful because I know so much more about me and people, me and circumstances, me and me. I am glad that I still have enough time to put this knowledge to good use.

From this journal entry, it appears that I started the midlife journey on a positive note. But over the last six or seven years I've sensed a slow, steady list left of center. Since the big four-o, I have had my share of startling "mirror moments"—times when my current reflection depresses me, compared against last year's Christmas picture. At times I have felt disheartened about growing older and have wrestled with God for perspective. I know what I *should* do, how I *should* feel; but most things in our culture do nothing to encourage me. I've read and listened to many strong, wise older women as they've shared about the joys of "moving on up there." But some days, quite honestly, I just don't want to get old. I have fears of fizzling out before I've made my contribution to the world—whatever it might be.

The Only Clock Worth Watching

I'm coming to believe that one of the secrets to aging well is lodged in our view of eternity. Some years after Christ's resurrection the apostle Paul wrote, "Since, then, you have been raised with Christ, set your hearts on things above....not on earthly things" (Col. 3:1–2). I don't take this to mean, "Keep your head in the clouds." Instead I hear, "Now you are spiritually programmed. Yes, you still breathe earth air. But the new, true you has begun functioning at a purer, higher altitude. So start thinking, talking, and acting like one who possesses *forever*."

Paul also encourages us with this: "Therefore we do not lose heart. Though outwardly we are wasting away, yet inwardly we are being renewed day by day....So we fix our eyes not on what is seen, but on what is unseen. For what is seen is temporary, but what is unseen is eternal" (2 Cor. 4:16, 18).

According to the Bible, since the day I gave my life to Christ, my heart has been hitched to eternity. There is no beginning, middle, or end to me now. All natural chronology has ceased. Though I live on a calendar-run globe, the real, true me is now perpetually, unceasingly timeless.

We may be getting older, but it's not too late for us to lock on to the concept of "forever" and erase from our cliché file phrases like, "I'm twenty-nine and holding," or, "I'm fifty-nine going on...well, let's just leave it at that." In a couple of months (it's good for me to practice saying this) I will be forty-seven earth-years old. I can hide this fact or mope about it. Or I can eternalize it.

This year I may try a new strategy. When someone asks, "How old are you?" I think I'll smile and say, "Actually…I'm infinity."

A little weird, I know. But just maybe I'll get to hear back, "Well, you sure look great for your age."

I give them eternal life, and they shall never perish; no one can snatch them out of my hand. (John 10:28)

🔳🔳 In the Chat Room

Martha, 49: *"I like my age, because I'm still young enough to do lots of things and enjoy my family—without feeling quite as tied down and responsible for them. I feel more laid back."*

Susan, 49: *"I love my age! I know where I'm creative and what I'm gifted to do. I also know what areas and situations are 'not me' and lead to frustration."*

Cathy, 42: *"Both my mother and grandmother died at fifty-eight. Now I see that age as quite young, and it's rather sobering."*

Suzie, 52: *"I started being aware of my changing body, emotions, and attitude around the age of thirty-eight. Weight gain began in my early forties. This year—my fifty-second—has been the most difficult one to adjust to. I think the key is humor. You have to laugh at all the dumb things you do and not get so serious about this season. My emotions are stronger now. I'm not as prone to cry. And I promised my family I would not bring any deadly weapons into the house!"*

Lauren, 44: *"I like my age mostly. It just sounds weird saying it out loud."*

June, 59: *"My fifty-second year was a doozy! I went through a huge crisis of grieving my fading youthfulness. Now I'm on the other side of it, and I truly love my life. The pressure is gone to look good for others. It's so freeing! I have only one true purpose now: to grow closer to Jesus. Midlife can't touch that or take it away."*

Pat, 49: *"I don't think about my age too much, except when my daughter reminds me. In my mind I'm still twenty-nine...Okay, maybe thirty-nine. If I didn't have so many physical symptoms telling me otherwise, I'd still believe I was thirty-nine! Sadly our culture treats aging with contempt, almost as if life itself is over. I refuse to accept this and plan to make a difference with my life."*

Putting the Crunch on Those Numbers

This year, don't let your birthday sneak up on you. Mark your calendar in bold letters and prepare to celebrate. Here are a few things to try:

- Spend part of the day enjoying yourself—by yourself. Do something you like to do but don't get the chance to do often. Pull out your sketchpad and draw by the lake or snap on your roller blades. Do something with your hair. Risk a new style or try highlights. Celebrate your body with a pedicure or massage, or get dressed up and have your picture taken. Buy a good book or magazine and read at an outdoor café or have a picnic in a lush city park.

- Challenge yourself to compliment as many people that day as there are candles on your cake. And *do* put candles on your cake. Celebrate every one. You've earned them!

- Call someone who would not expect to hear from you and tell them how they've impacted your life.

- Write out three personal goals you'd like to accomplish by your next birthday. Tell someone else. Keep these goals where you can see them.

- Be bold and plan your own birthday party! (Bonus points if you can make it a surprise.) Buy your favorite flowers. Wear your favorite outfit. Play your favorite music. Serve your favorite foods. Enjoy your favorite friends. If you have home movies or videos, run them on mute in the background. Display your yearbooks and photos. At some point pull all of your guests together and count your blessings aloud to them—one blessing for each year of your life.

- Record your history. Author Carolyn Warner writes, "Preparing your own chronological chart is an excellent tool....Prepare it in five-year increments beginning from your birth. In an opposite column, list three or four significant things that happened (in the world) during each five-year period."[1] You might also want to list family and personal milestones. A shorter version: Draw a timeline of your life, divide it into ten-year increments, then give a title or label to each decade. Keep your chart or timeline in a scrapbook or photo album.

Midlife Awareness Quiz

For optimal success in any new culture, it's always a good idea to become familiar with the key phrases and terms unique to that locale. To help gauge your readiness for the journey ahead, grab a pen and take this quick and easy Midlife Awareness Quiz. Feel free to consult whatever avenues of information you have at your disposal. NOTE: You cannot fail this quiz. Read each question carefully, then draw a line under the answer you like best.

1. *A* mammogram *is:*
   □ A message from your mother delivered to your front door
   □ A nutritional cracker designed for nursing moms
   □ A heaping unit of measure used in baking biscuits in the South
   □ A cruel but vital test to measure a woman's threshold of pain

2. *If a woman has her bunions removed, she has:*
   □ Asked her server to clear the remains of a fried Australian appetizer
   □ Paid for posterior liposuction
   □ Loosed her hair from its bun-dage
   □ Just returned from a great shoe sale

3. *The word* midlife *comes from:*
   □ A little known novel by J. R. R. Tolkien
   □ A Midland, Texas, church choir newsletter
   □ A seventeenth-century saint often arrested for sudden, disturbing outbursts
   □ A forty-something lexicographer in denial

4. *The term* middle-age spread *refers to:*
   □ A margarine product for people over forty
   □ A chic trend in bed linens designed from ancient fabrics
   □ A dude ranch turned weight-loss clinic in central Wyoming
   □ The trunk region of a mature body storing excess fat to protect vital organs

5. *When a woman is in menopause, she is:*
   □ Taking an afternoon nap

☐ Pressing the stop button on an IBM copier
☐ Taking a break from the Dictaphone
☐ Free to do whatever she wants—any day of the month—for the rest of her life

6. *The abbreviation HRT stands for:*
☐ Handsome Research Technician
☐ Holy Redeemer Tabernacle
☐ Humor Replacement Therapy
☐ Hoping for a Reduction in Temperature

7. *When someone says they have an empty nest, they really mean:*
☐ A zero-balance retirement account
☐ The post atop the mast of a ship
☐ The code name for an abandoned spy hideout
☐ Clean, quiet housing for dazed and recovering parents

8. *The best definition of a hot flash is:*
☐ A popular Web site for late-breaking news
☐ The time between listing your teen's chores and his or her disappearance
☐ A new urban street dance done with flashlights
☐ A single surge of power reported to burn three hundred calories per second and heat the entire town of Hooterville for fifteen minutes

9. *When someone gets bifocals, that person can:*
☐ Enter a two-man Olympic archery event
☐ Easily learn how to multitask
☐ Sing in two octaves at once
☐ Help you read the dinner menu

10. *If a midlife woman says she has lost weight, she:*
☐ Has spent too long in a checkout line
☐ Has misplaced her workout equipment
☐ Has important papers blowing across her desk
☐ Has witnessed an outright miracle

PART 2

Ch-ch-ch-ch-changes

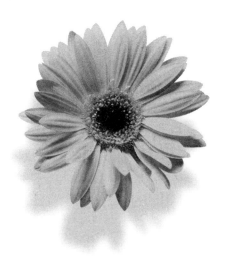

6

Whoever thought up the word
mammogram? Every time I hear it,
I think I'm supposed to put my
breast in an envelope and
send it to someone.
—Jan King

In Defense of the Chicken-Breasted Mammogram

Some people have a strong aversion to medical procedures. Nothing against medical professionals, it's just that certain people get paranoid when it comes to exams of a potentially painful or exploratory nature. They are more afraid of piercing needles and snappy gloves than all the world's cancer, heart disease, and flesh-eating bacteria combined.

I happen to be a charter member of this group. And that's one of the arguments I've used to put off getting a mammogram...for seven years now.

For Shame!

I know. According to the American Medical Association, the American Cancer Society, and every breast cancer patient in the world, my (lack of) action is unthinkable. But aside from being a natural-born chicken, I've rationalized this negligence with several other impressive lines of reasoning:

- I am a healthy person. I feel fine. Why go fishing for trouble?

- I keep intending to do it but can never find a good time.

- Arranging appointments is a hassle. It's: Find a date that works for you and the doctor. Carve out half a day. Get the initial exam. Then, prescription in hand, call for the mammogram appointment. Carve out another half a day. You know the drill.

- I don't especially care for strangers, officially certified or not, gawking and poking in places they don't belong.

- Mammograms can hurt. I have witnesses and sworn statements to prove this.

- When a girl has spent her entire life dodging discomfort, she is not about to pay a health-care professional to give it to inflict it upon her.

I realize that to someone staring at surgical scars, these excuses sound pathetically lame. But at one time or another, they have given me the perfect smoke screen for denial. I say "denial" because everyone knows that a mammogram is a serious rite of passage, a coming-of-middle-age must-do; and when a woman gets one, she clearly and forever crosses over to the far side. Officially she becomes one of "them." That means the longer she puts it off, the longer she is able to trick herself into thinking she is younger than all those other women her age.

Diary of a Mammogram

But now, in the interest of journalistic research, I have decided to get a mammogram despite the obvious risk of mutilation. My plan is to bring you along for accountability and moral support. I'm also hoping that by offering a little play-by-play, color commentary of my experience, those sisters among us who remain closed-chested to the idea might somehow be inspired to follow suit.

(Note: No part of the following account has been fictionalized not even a little).

9:00 A.M. Thursday, March 14

It is the morning of my first mammogram. Before leaving home I do the essential bathing and trimming, dress in a two-piece outfit, and forgo my antiperspirant as instructed. Why we are forbidden to wear deodorant, one can only speculate. On the way out the door, I pop a few over-the-counter pain relievers to take off the anticipated edge. (Every little bit helps.)

My destination is Celebration Hospital, near Disney World. I chose this site because a TV special on mammograms reported on a new technique that looks something like an ultrasound, is supposedly better at early detection, and involves next-to-no pain. After quizzing my gynecologist about it (we do not feel it is in your best interest to reveal how long it had been since my last pap smear), I learned that Celebration Hospital is one of a few places in the country with the very latest mammography equipment. So, being the glutton for gridlocked tourist traffic that I am, I drive off in that direction.

9:45 A.M. Hospital Disney-Style

Walking in Celebration Hospital reception area looks more like a grand hotel than a place to fix sick people. At the desk a very nice lady gives me a beeper and tells me to have a seat. On one side of the atrium is a giant video wall showing a movie of vibrant fall leaves reflecting in a stream. It's like a water prism—a liquid impressionist painting put to acoustic guitar. I admire the camera work and the creative people who thought to seep calm into this atmosphere where fidgety, over-forty women wait for their first mammograms.

9:50 A.M. That'll Be One Hundred Dollars, Please

The beeper goes off, and I'm directed to a woman in the finance office. This is a quiet room, without the usual ranting over unpaid bills standard in such places. As I study what looks like a postcard of an ancient harem on her desk, the woman asks me for one hundred dollars. *One hundred dollars!* It's not that I don't have the money; it's just that I've never had to come up with this large a co-pay before. (No wonder we put these things off.)

After handing over my credit card, the finance person asks to see my insurance card too. This is slightly annoying, for two reasons: (1) I already spent thirty minutes on the phone the other day dispensing this information to "central bookkeeping," and (2) the card in question has been lost ever since I gave it to one of my sons who says he's really sorry but cannot find it and maybe it's in a pants pocket that might be—surprise, surprise—somewhere near the base of the Tower of T-Shirt Terror in his bedroom.

10:05 A.M. Entering the Imaging Center

Upstairs at the entrance to the imaging center there is a man (of all people) sitting behind a decorative, concierge-looking desk. Secretly I decided that he's probably assigned to this post in case one of us tries to go AWOL. The man checks my name off a roster then hands me a letter from his boss, who would like me to know about the various types of mammograms available at this facility.

Just as I start to read, Rose appears.

Rose is a chirpy senior citizen who has come to lead me to my doom. As we navigate the halls, I ask how long she's been working here. "About two months," she tells me, "just while I've been on vacation." Rose comes to Orlando every winter, and when I ask why a woman on vacation would want to volunteer in a hospital, she answers, "Oh, I just like helping people." (I would like to be able to say that I would give this exact same answer twenty years from now, but at the moment all I can picture is David and me lounging on a beach in the tropics, slurping frozen fruit drinks.)

Arriving at our destination, Rose offers me a front-open gown, says good-bye, and heads back for the next victim.

10:10 A.M. Putting My Best Chest Forward

Top off, gown on, I enter a low-lit room so a woman named Sylvia can get more information. She wants to know my age, my age when I had my first child, if I smoke, and if anyone on my mother's side has had breast cancer. I say an aunt on my father's side had surgery, but she waves this off. We're only concerned with maternal lines. "And how long since your last mammogram?" she asks. "Well...this would be my first," I say, then brace for a scalding lecture that never comes.

In front of a mirror, Sylvia schools me in the art of the standing self-exam. Arms down, arms up, shoulders forward, check the collarbone, side view, hands on hips. "Breasts are at their most normal state about ten days after our periods," she says, "so try to do this every month at that time."

But what if you miss a few inches? How can you feel a tiny tumor with all this fatty tissue throwing you off? Besides, no matter when I do a home exam, I always feel lumps. "You should know your breasts," she says. "You should be so familiar with them that it's easy to tell when something's out of place."

You would think after forty-seven years, this would not be a problem.

At one point Sylvia asks if a certain section feels tender and I say, "Some." She writes that down and draws a circle on a breast diagram on her clipboard. I know from a TV special that the area she has circled is the most frequent spot for breast cancer. But I am not worried, and she doesn't flinch. This is the first day of my period; tissues are sore. She feels a similar place on the other side and makes a note of that too.

10:15 A.M. The Torture Chamber

The machine in front of me turns out not to be the ultrasound version I had hoped for but looks like the dreaded, breast-maiming kind I've heard about. This confuses me, but the young female technician has already moved into gear, so I keep quiet. According to the TV special, this is what you do *not* do. You are supposed to take charge of your mammograms. But the girl seems so sweet that I go like a pig to the slaughter.

Easing me up to the edge of a gray "plate," she fixes my flesh like a baker with his dough. She is careful but firm, and, to my surprise, this does not bother me.

Apparently this is my lucky day, because the new digital machine she is using is only FDA approved for "smaller cup sizes." In a few months they expect similar technology for larger busts, but right now only small-busted women get this special treatment. From what I understand, my photos will be "exceptional digital quality," ready for viewing in only ten seconds.

10:19 A.M. No Turning Back

Behind a partition, my new bosom buddy hits a switch, and a clear, acrylic tray clamps down on my breast. I look straight ahead and think of the comments of my sister and others who had traumatic first experiences. I clinch my hand into a fist, hoping to fool the pain. The girl pumps something hydraulic-sounding, and the tray presses down further. Again, more pressure. Then one last time for the whole enchilada. "Hold your breath," she says, "hold, hoooooooold." Then *whoosh*, the pressure lifts, and she tells me to breathe.

Hmmm. Not too bad. Some discomfort, but still a ways from excruciating.

Now for side B. More flailing and flopping of skin in the manner of play dough. Then comes the pressure again. It's tight. Tiiiiighter. "Now hold your breath, hold, hoooooooold. Now breathe."

My gosh…is that it?

No, there are two more. (*This* must be when you die.) The side views are awkward. There's a pinch under my arm, but nothing I need to *take charge* of. The technician has me tilt my head and hold it there. It's a lovely pose, perfect for *Mammogram Monthly*.

10:25 A.M. It Is Finished

Two more times I hold my breath, and in only eight, ten minutes tops, the whole ordeal is over.

I want to hug this girl, buy her expensive gifts, name a street after her, but instead I stay composed and steal a glance at the slate-and-white-veined negative of my mammaries on the computer screen. No obvious, glaring clots, but since I've never seen one of these before, I have no idea how to read it. I want the girl to say what, if anything, she sees. But even though these are my pictures, I am not assertive because I know the standard answer: "I don't read them; I just take them." The girl is nice but neutral. No stricken voice, dilated pupils, or gasps usually associated with the sudden evidence of catastrophic disease, so I take this as a good sign.

"You should get the results in about a week," she says.

Then I thank her (Did I say *thank* her?) put on my top, fluff my hair, and let myself out.

10:40 A.M. Damage Assessment

Back in my car, I take emotional inventory. There is relief that I, total queen of the lily-livered, was somehow spared the trauma experienced by others less fortunate. I feel sheepish and silly for so long avoiding what turned out to be such a simple exercise. And instead of feeling like I thought I would—as if I had been inducted into the Aged Matrons Club—it just may be that I sense a hint of empowerment.

A Bible verse that has always intrigued me says, "You are [Sarah's] daughters if you do what is right and do not give way to fear" (1 Pet. 3:6). We know that Sarah was an aging nomad, the wife of Abraham, who was often placed in perilous situations. Her destiny always seemed hazy, but this fact didn't seem to rattle her.

In this verse God hails Sarah—applauds her. He singles her out in history. Why? Because in times of dry-mouthed anxiety, she managed to stay her pioneering course. So impressed was God with this that he goes out of his way to exhort all his girls to live likewise.

If there is any certainty about midlife, it's that we now face plenty of uncertainty. And it's here that we're in league with Sarah.

As I continue up the interstate, two thoughts occur to me. First, if today is any indication, middle age—for all the hype about its treacherous, untried territories—may just prove to be a fair, hospitable land. And second, wisdom would dictate that I head for some antiperspirant—pronto.

(Note: Both pap smear and mammogram were pronounced normal.)

Search me, O God, and know my heart; test me and know my anxious thoughts. (Ps. 139:23)

In the Chat Room

Shirley, 40: *"When it was time for my first mammogram, my mother was so worried about how I'd feel that she offered to go with me. But the whole experience was a piece of cake. I think the fact that I'd been off caffeine for two years may have helped."*

Lauren, 44: *"My mammograms are no fun. They can't get everything in, so they have to repeat it over and over."*

Julie, 39: *"My first mammogram was so traumatic and painful that after it was over, I dropped to my knees and fainted. The technician said she'd never seen anyone do that before."*

53

Martha, 49: *"One of my mammograms was at an imaging center where I had never been before. They saw something on the screen that had always been there and kept redoing one side. After making a pancake of it and scaring me with biopsy suggestions, I finally asked them to look at my previous mammograms. They did and said, 'Oh, never mind.' That was somewhat of a pain."*

For Procrastinators

If you are putting off getting your first mammogram, here are some suggestions:

- Try to get at the real roots of why you are procrastinating.

- Talk to at least five women who have had mammograms. Ask for tips to make the experience easier, and get recommendations for the best imaging center in your area.

- Read the most current literature you can find on mammography.

- Give yourself a deadline. Make an appointment and stick the date on the refrigerator, or write it in bold in your organizer. Don't cancel! Ask a friend or family member to keep you accountable. Or better yet, have the person go with you.

- Talk with a nurse, doctor, or even a breast-cancer patient if months go by and you are still putting it off.

- Do it for someone you love.

Trust me. If I can do it, you can do it.

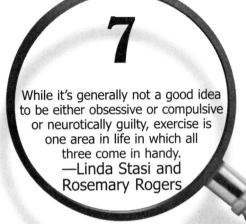

7

While it's generally not a good idea to be either obsessive or compulsive or neurotically guilty, exercise is one area in life in which all three come in handy.
—Linda Stasi and Rosemary Rogers

Huffin' with the Health-Club Hotties

Some people pop right out of bed each morning, anxious to go for a quick, invigorating jog. To be totally honest, I would rather clean toilets than exercise—even though it does promise a nice endorphin high for all the sweat you have to go through to get it. At my age, however, I feel I no longer have a choice in the matter. It's pretty much do or dilapidate. Which is why David and I joined a health club.

Even if we haven't always practiced healthful living, since the midseventies we have been big believers in the benefits of exercise. So when a new fitness club went up just a block from our house, we decided it was time to invest in a healthy future.

The only requirements were a minor membership fee: two years slave labor, and a pledge of all our home equity for security.

Our new club is not one of those wholesale workout warehouses or flab-friendly YMCAs. As luck (or providence?) would have it, it's a brand-new, state-of-the-art, full-service health facility. Professional athletes train there, along with a few other famous people (although we've never actually seen them). Even the more regular members are not your average gym club tire-kickers. They are spit-in-your-hand, let's-heave-some-weight-around kick-boxer types whose primary mission in life is to one day make the cover of *Bulging Body Beautiful* magazine.

Mama Cass Meets Twiggy

My first trip to the club revealed that I was in deep fitness weeds. Not one woman in the whole building was above a size 4, and only 2 percent of the population appeared to be over twenty-five. Showing up in your sorry-excuse-for-workout clothes is bad enough, but walk in a place like this packing a few extra pounds, and you're asking for self-image suicide!

Whenever I go slinking around the weight machines, pretending to know how they work, it's hard not to stare at the cute, ripped girls who fiercely focus on their muscle sculpting routines. They're such a curious marvel. How do they get that inhuman power to turn down cheesecake and pasta? Do they have any idea that their thighs never touch, even when they sit down? Where can I go to buy whatever they've got that makes a woman show up at the gym every single day, whether she wants to or not?

One elite group of primo-talented girls at this club really blows me away. Imagine this: There I am, gasping my lungs out, walking a sprightly 3.5 miles per hour on the treadmill, and to my left I see a tiny, no-fat sweetheart who is going to town on her elliptical machine—and chatting away on her cell phone. I can't think straight, much less talk straight, and here this girl is having a long, highly animated conversation (in which she seems to be doing all the talking). Minutes later the girl on the treadmill to my right opens up a textbook and reads while running at a five-mile-an-hour pace. How is this possible? I have walked on treadmills while trying, with great effort, to scan large, full page magazine photos, but that's about the best I can do.

If you've ever been on a treadmill, you know it requires a certain degree of agility. Several times I have found myself going at a pretty good clip when, without warning, I suddenly clunked off the back of the machine onto the floor. People pretend not to see, but you know they have to be snickering. When this horror happens to you, all you can do is pick up your shell-shocked self and *chassé jeté* for the rotating ramp like a cowboy mounting his trick horse.

It's not that I'm uncoordinated. It's just that it's easy to ride right off the edge of one of these contraptions when your attention is locked on more important things—like breathing, watching the goings on of skinny people, and squinting to read the closed captioning on the TV hanging from the ceiling.

The real kicker comes one day as I'm straining to do my squats. There I am, clinching my five-pound hand weights, when I glance up and see a petite young thing doing a long series of lunges across the floor in the aerobics room while (you guessed it) talking a mile a minute on her cell phone. I can only think of one explanation for this kind of extreme behavior: a new fitness craze called Phone-A-Coach in which unseen instructors talk people through their workouts from an undisclosed location.

You're probably wondering at this point why I bother with the health club at all. How much ego-bashing can one woman take? More than once it has come to my attention that I am the largest female athlete there. This is a miserable revelation—like being dressed in a formal at the company picnic. It sometimes adds fuel to my dread of daily workouts.

But whatever the price to my ego, the club does have its advantages. For example, David and I can work out together several times a week. There's a variety of equipment and classes to choose from if a particular routine gets boring. All the weight machines I'll ever need are in one place, just waiting to build the muscles that are supposed to burn all this fat and strengthen my bones. And if it's true that you become like the people you associate with, then just maybe a bit of the dedication and drive I see in the girls there will someday latch on to me.

How in the World Did We Get Here?

Have you ever seen a Body Mass Index (BMI) table? It's a shocker of a tool that looks like the chart on the back of your hosiery package. It helps you determine (in case you're not sure) if you are underweight, "weight appropriate," overweight, or obese. The other day I located my weight and height on one of those BMI tables and discovered that because I weigh (what I weigh) and I'm five-foot-four, I am one gray square away from *obese*. How is this possible?

If you have ever struggled with weight issues, you've probably come up with a few reasons to explain your excess poundage. Here are some of mine:

- I am forty-seven years old.

- I come from a family of molasses-slow metabolizers.

- I am near menopause, which further slows a metabolism that only dynamite could budge.

- I am a writer—the worst possible eaters' profession—which means that sometimes I sit for days and weeks at a time (like I am doing right now), only moving to eat, sleep, and throw things at my computer.

- All my life I have been a "stress eater" addicted to carbohydrates. I admit I seek comfort in food.

There were seasons in the past when I ran three miles a day, kept my weight down, and had lots of energy. Then my knee gave out, my schedule changed, I had a crisis or two, and we moved a few times. You know how it is. Before too long you're too out of shape to reel yourself back in line.

Once you get past a certain number on the scale, it's easy to live in denial about how bad things really are. For a while I refused to weigh myself, thinking I would be less obsessed with my weight if I tried concentrating on my clothing size. This tactic works for some, but it didn't work for me. The weight kept inching up until it was easy to excuse going up one size here, another there—because, after all, everyone knows certain brands are cut differently.

Over My Deadly Body

Much has been said and written about learning to accept our bodies, about loving and blessing ourselves as we are. This is a good principle. It's helped many women to break the vicious cycle of body-hate and depression and stop putting off happiness. But here's where I must voice some caution.

At the moment I love my "soul" self, but the rest of me is not acting in my best interest. There is too much evidence about the damaging downsides of weight gain for me to feel good about continuing to pamper this porky, puffy person.

In her book *The Wisdom of Menopause*, Dr. Christiane Northrup highlights some of those downsides. "A 1999 study from Harvard Medical School," she writes, "found that women who gain approximately twenty pounds in adulthood experience a decline in physical function and vitality even greater than that associated with smoking."[1] (Yikes!) She also says, "Abdominal fat cells are more metabolically active…and potentially more dangerous than fat cells on your hips and thighs. They can contribute to insulin resistance (as in diabetes)…and they can pump out too much androgen (as in male hormones) and estrogen (as in hotter hot flashes)."[2]

Given these and other informed warnings on the complications of excess weight, it's hard for me to view my jiggly thighs and torso as objects to pet, coddle, and love. Right now they're more like deadly weapons.

I know man looks on the outward appearance, and God looks on the heart. I am confident that God loves me unconditionally; head to toe, as I am. But here's a question: If such great care was taken in Old Testament times to build and maintain God's tabernacle, how much more should I care for my body, which is God's living, holy temple?

My Body, God's Billboard

My desire is to reflect the house of my Master, Jesus Christ, with as much visible excellence as I'm capable of. Not perfection by a long stretch. Not cover-girl false or beanpole thin, achieved by devoting hours a day to my flesh. But I do want to represent Christ with energy and enthusiasm. I want to be maximum for him, healthy enough to help people in a quality way for as many years as possible. And if I can help it, I don't want to create a stumbling block for someone who might reject God's message through me because of their bias against bigness.

We should be kind to ourselves, yes, and never judgmental or Pharisaical about anyone else's eating habits or body type. But we also need to love ourselves enough to dig up the emotional (or medical) roots that keep us trapped in habitual, negative food patterns year after year. We should be patient with ourselves through the process and ask for help. But if weight is a problem, we need to act now.

For women our age, exercise is not an option if we ever hope to:

- Burn fat (and wear a swimsuit again)

- Build muscle to trick our possum-playing metabolism into burning even more fat

- Lessen (maybe even lose) some pesky perimenopausal symptoms

- Strengthen those bones everyone is so worried about

- Clear up our adult acne

- Reduce the production of unfeminine androgens

- Improve our emotional outlook

- Increase our stamina

- And enjoy a long, fruitful life

I don't know about you, but I want to be able to walk into a room with no thought of my size. I want to welcome cameras (at any angle), warm weather, sleeveless blouses, and my patient, affectionate husband. I want to beat this weight thing, once and for all, this year. And if you want, you can help keep me accountable by contacting me at www.caronloveless.com and asking how the weight loss is going.

Huffin' with the health-club hotties has been hard—okay, some days, downright depressing. I won't ever look like those girls, and it's highly unlikely that I will ever become an exercise addict. But God is using the women at my health club—without their saying a word—to challenge me to better health and motivate me to want to restore the original wrapper he programmed in me. Their drive and discipline speak to me, saying, "Make better choices." "Don't give up." "Consistency will make a difference." And, "We'll see you back here tomorrow...but you might want to do something about that T-shirt."

In the Chat Room

Lisa, 47: "If I could change anything, it would be to tone up and lose a little weight, which seems to have settled in my middle body. I don't like that. I've always been thin till now."

Martha, 49: "I wish I'd taken better care of my health when I was younger. Too little sleep, too much stress, and too much junk food in my twenties and thirties have caused my body to age quicker. I used to feel I could push myself to keep going nonstop. Now I feel tired and drained when I don't take care of myself. It's harder to lose weight, and I can't stay up late like I used to."

Karen, 65: "I'm not a size 12 anymore. It's 14 and sometimes 16. I'm not willing to do what it takes to be slimmer. I'm not concerned enough."

Patricia, 49: "I will never have the hard body of a twenty-year-old. I guess I could, if I were willing to put the hours and work into it. I have accumulated some padding—'fat' seems too harsh—that I would like to tone. It does bother me a little bit."

June, 59: *"I try to look past the exterior and not focus on my physical self so much. I actually find myself happier when I keep my focus off 'self' and on others. Self-image is just not that important anymore."*

No, I beat my body and make it my slave so that after I have preached to others, I myself will not be disqualified for the prize. (1 Cor. 9:27)

Where to Gain Help If You're Ready to Lose

If you could stand to lose a few pounds (or more) and are ready to do something about it, here are some resources to try:

www.pamsmith.com—I mentioned Pam's Web site in chapter 5. What I didn't tell you is that, in addition to being a well-known nutritionist, she is an energy coach to professional athletes, a best-selling author, and a great friend of mine. Click on her Web site for books, tapes, and other materials that can help you with proper eating, weight loss, and living well.

Fight Fat after Forty by Pamela Peeke, M.D., M.P.H.

Weight Stages: Successfully Manage Your Weight through Life's Ups and Downs by Weight Watchers.

8

Refuse to think of them
as chin hairs. Think of them
as stray eyebrows.
—Janette Barber

Keeping Your
Chin Up

Throughout history there have been strange sightings of hair on regions of a woman's body typically associated with the male gender. I *have* seen a few girls with mustaches. And I will admit that once in the last year I actually toyed with the idea of using my husband's battery-operated nose clippers. But where was I when they issued the warning on chin hair?

Maybe the girls you hang out with openly discuss this sort of thing, but for some reason, my circle was a bit hush-hush on this topic. And I never had a grandmother who said, "Honey, one day you will be minding your own business, freshening your lipstick, when suddenly you'll see spikes the size of broom straws poking out your chin. But don't be alarmed. It's just the first wave of the change."

Uninvited chin hair can be quite a shock to a girl. It lumps you right in there with Colonel Sanders, Abraham Lincoln, and the Three Little Pigs. Leg stubble we understand. But it can be a real out-of-body experience going chin-to-chin with your fifteen-year-old son and winning by unanimous decision. Trust me, I know.

Therefore, as a public service to women everywhere who are still clueless about the formidable foe that may be lurking just beneath their moisturizer, I will attempt to share the small bit of light I have been forced to gather on this subject.

A Routine Change

For more years than I care to count, the start of my day has consisted of visiting the various stations of the bathroom in a certain predictable order. That routine is no longer possible. Now, immediately upon waking, my most urgent business is to run to the magnifying mirror and rid myself of any new "evidence" that has cropped up overnight.

In the beginning I noticed random patches of peach fuzz, and a quick patrol of the affected area was all that was required. But over time the little rascals regrouped and came back with reinforcements. In order to avoid a full-scale invasion, my only course of action has been to march into the bathroom first thing in the morning and pluck them out with a passion similar to that of a wild, rabid gardener yanking weeds.

If you haven't reached this stage yet, you need to prepare yourself for the reality that dislodging every last one of these intruders can take a large chunk of time—due in part (if you are anywhere in the vicinity of thirty-nine) to your eyes not being as fit as they once were. And I don't know about you, but I can't afford to prolong my already generous occupation of the lavatory.

In fact, we should probably agree here and now that one hour is about the maximum legal limit an average-size woman should spend on beautification. In that time we are called on to shower, shampoo, shave, dry, spritz, smear, dab, conceal, blend, brush, snip, squeeze, try on, discard, try on again, style, shine, poof, spray, and work any number of cosmetic miracles common to all artistically-enhanced women. That's quite a workout. Therefore, one full hour—though it's max—is pretty well justified. Any more than that, and we might as well set up office hours.

(Note: If the only pair of tweezers you own is the one you used to pull splinters out of your child's feet ten years ago, discard it. Hair removal of this nature falls just short of minor surgery. Buy the most expensive brand you can afford. I got mine—"Tweezerman"—at the drugstore for about fourteen dollars.)

How Hair Happens

At a time like this, a question worth asking might be, "Why do so many middle-age women grow auxiliary hair in the first place?" According to Dr. John Lee in his book *What Your Doctor May Not Tell You about Premenopause*, excess hair growth usually occurs because a woman's hormone-manufacturing plant has begun releasing a potent little product called *androstenedione* (better known to us in the South as a "male hormone").

If this is news to you, brace yourself. Apparently this male hormone is kin to the one that was responsible for putting hair on your nephew's chest and lowering his voice an octave. And when your batch of androstenedione gets loose, the same thing could happen to you.

Wait, there's more. Not only can a woman in the throes of midlife develop overactive glands and follicles; she can also get male-pattern baldness, a bulging midriff, and her face, chest, and back can begin to expand to more masculine proportions. (And here I was panicked about hot flashes.) The proper medical term for this manifestation, according to Dr. Lee, is being *andro-genic*, which is something you can learn more about at your local library or health-food store if you have a feeling this condition may apply to someone in your immediate family.

In the event this whole hair thing gets really out of hand, you will have no recourse but to join the millions of baby-booming women who laser, wax, or pay total strangers to shock them in the face with electric needles on a monthly basis.

Here's the Point

I've found that renegade hair, like other midlife experiences, is good for exposing a woman's most private anxieties. It confirms one of our worst fears: that our bodies are growing a mind of their own. No longer can we fully count on them to be there for us.

These days I am standing in the foyer of midlife, watching the door to What Was close behind me; and part of me, if I'm honest, feels cheated sometimes. Even though I've been given so much, I find myself acting like the child who gets a dollar bill from her daddy every day for a week and then pitches a fit the next week when all he has to give is fifty cents.

If we're going to make the most of these new, foreign experiences—if we're going to get some good mileage out of them—we've got to find ways to translate them into a language our souls understand. It's easy to look in the mirror and obsess about the changing face of our lives. It's more challenging to get still enough to listen and understand what the God Who Never Changes is trying to say to us through it.

If we let them, even the smallest of midlife issues can bring a new level of clarity. They can help us sort through what's important *now*. They have the power to say, "No, it isn't your imagination. The nights *are* getting cooler. The days *are* getting shorter. And by the looks of things, there's a pretty good chance you already have used up more than half the days you're scheduled for. So be all the more vigilant not to squander the rest."

Okay, so I missed the memo on chin hair. Now that it has shown up for the party, I plan to put it to work. I want it to be a sign to me. I want it to say that the evidence is clear: There is no time to waste on lesser things. As I look in the mirror each morning, I want it to cause me to think: *Be fully here for your husband. Be fully alive for your sons. Show up for your life today—and hold nothing back!*

Walk while you have the light. (John 12:35)

☞ ☞ In the Chat Room

Mimi, 42: *"I was in the car with my ten-year-old, and she said, 'Mom, there's a hair sticking out of your chin.' I glanced in the rearview mirror and said, 'Where? I don't see it.' Then she said, 'No, look on your other chin.'"*

Lu Anne, 37: *"All I want to know is, what's with the back fat? Where did that come from—and all the unwanted hair? I wasn't ready for this."*

Linda, 37: *"Not long ago a good friend of mine came over, plopped on the couch, and said, 'I've got to know something. What is the deal with these nipple hairs? This can't be normal.' When I screamed, 'Ohmygosh! You have those too?' we both just couldn't stop laughing."*

Tante, 51: *"One of my patients said she no longer has to shave because the hair under her arms and legs stopped growing. However, hair is now growing on her chin and upper lip."*

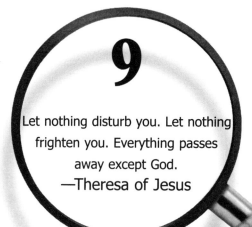

Let nothing disturb you. Let nothing frighten you. Everything passes away except God.
—Theresa of Jesus

When Little Fears Become a Factor

As a rule I'm not a fearful person. I don't mind traveling alone. I'm not particularly scared of bugs. Nor do planes or public speaking make me nervous. But lately I've caught wind of some new, subtle fears trying to sneak in the back door and raid the place. Maybe some of them have left footprints at your house too.

The Footprints of Fear

Here are four that, for me, are particularly persistent:

1. Fear of amnesia

This one jabs me below the belt sometimes when I teach or

speak. I've been getting up in front of groups for over twenty years, and in that time I've developed a degree of comfortability in communicating. But these days I get concerned that I will lose my train of thought or forget a point I'm trying to make. I'm afraid to trust my memory, so I rely much more on my notes.

I worry that I'll be speaking and suddenly realize (as happened recently) that the word I intended to say did not make it out, but something else did—perhaps something God wished to say to those with Gaelic ancestry. These days such a thing can happen with no warning. Just *splat,* and out it comes. Not long ago I was giving the announcements in one of our church services, and I said something like this: "If you're a guest with us today, we're thrilled that you're here. And if you would take just a moment to open your *wbatham,* I-I-I'd like to walk you through…." I have a theory that when this happens to me, I am actually in the middle of some kind of micro-ministroke—but I am not yet prepared for you to quote me on that.

Another delightful experience I've had more than once is stopping midthought to see if someone in the audience can help me find the word I'm trying to use. I'll get stuck and say, "*You know,* it's that really tall metal thingy with the round deal on top. Has the name of the town written on it. You know, there's water inside? Like the one on Petticoat Junction. Okay, ten dollars to the first person who can tell me what I'm talking about." Along with incidents like these come "little voices" (usually during the wee hours) that question whether I've still got what it takes to be a good communicator.

This midlife amnesia seems to strike at the most inopportune moments. Because I'm a church staff member and pastor's wife, every week I meet new people who—you really can't fault them for this—would like me to know their names. Though I've never been great at name recall, I recently had a situation that shows just how bad things have become. After one of our services, a pretty twenty-one-year-old girl walked up and introduced herself to me. Turns out she is the daughter of the matron of honor in my wedding, whom I hadn't seen in over fifteen years. Not more than one sentence later, I had already forgotten her name. Right in the midst of our joyful reunion, I had to apologize and say, "I'm so sorry, honey. Please tell me your name again."

This problem is beginning to affect other important areas of my life—like shopping. Here's what happens: I see a woman at the other end of the grocery store aisle. I should know her name; our kids go to school together. But all that comes up on my mental monitor screen is a last name, so the best I can do when I pass her is to say, "Well, how are things with Mrs. Fizzlebaum today?" I would like to add, "I know you're only the mother of my son's best friend since kindergarten, but would you excuse me for a moment while I report some stolen brain cells?" More than once, I'm embarrassed to admit, I have sneaked my cart to the other end of the store, hoping to avoid this exact scenario.

2. Fear of abandonment

More than usual now, my mind wanders over to a whole slush pile of unpleasant possibilities. I find myself imagining what it will feel like when my husband is gone (assuming he goes before I do) or when my kids get so busy with their own families and careers that they have no time for me.

I think of the movie *Driving Miss Daisy* and remember how, as Miss Daisy got older, her son came to see her less and less. This kind of scenario is a hard one for me to navigate emotionally. I remember the responsibility/resentment battle I went through in the days when I had to keep up with my family, extended family, household chores, ministry responsibilities, and writing assignments, while also being available for a sick mom across town. I worry that the day will come when those same conflicting feelings surface in my adult children—when I become a "have-to" and a drain on their emotional gas tanks.

At the moment I am especially blessed. My husband is healthy, and my sons and daughter-in-law live at home or in the same town. But the odds that things will remain this way forever are low, and I wonder how I'll feel in twenty years. I can see me now: all sprawled out on the couch in an unwashed bathrobe, eating cheeseburgers and watching old black-and-white movies at two o'clock in the afternoon. I've battled depression before, and sometimes I worry that it will come back in a big way if I end up alone. Me, the one who jumps at the chance to lunch or shop by herself, who needs her space like others need their sleep!

3. Fear of Alzheimer's

My grandmother (and last remaining grandparent) has Alzheimer's disease and lives in a nursing home. She and I have similar builds, similar coloring, and although I've never told her this, similar easily agitated, nerve-sensitive colons. I'm not claiming to be a geneticist, but it does seem that a generous portion of my gene pool has been passed down from my grandmother. And more than a few times the thought has come to me that what has happened to her will probably happen to me.

I know next to nothing about Alzheimer's except that it can be hereditary, and at the moment, it is incurable. Now when I forget things, instead of thinking, *Oh, this is just the natural forgetfulness we all experience as we age*, I can't help but wonder if it's really some early-stage evidence that I have the disease.

4. Fear of the "fatal attraction"

Every wife probably has a few times in her marriage when she becomes aware of an attractive or aggressive or extra-attentive female hovering around her husband. And sometimes that flips a switch. This has happened to me. Rationally, sensibly, I know I have no logical reason to feel insecure. Still, on a few occasions, I've found myself grilling David over some innocent, random exchange he could barely remember. There has been no breach of trust in our past to give me grounds for feeling suspicious. David has done nothing wrong—except be in the right place at the wrong time, perhaps. Still, something sets me off. And suddenly my mind takes one plus three and turns it into twelve.

I hate when this happens. But once the fire is lit, it's hard to contain. Thankfully David has been patient, hearing my questions, letting me work through concerns, doing his best to uncover the source of what unsettles me. Typically the problem is something in me, not in him. In time my perspective tends to smooth out, and I see that I overreacted in the heat of what was probably another hormonally-charged moment.

Scaring Fear to Death

Taking the time to sit down and admit our random fears in writing is one way we can shine a flashlight in their eyes and force them to come out with their hands up. Whenever I do this, I am better able to recognize and deal with those fears more quickly the next time they arise.

Talking with other women helps too. In the midlife focus group I told you about in chapter 4, many women voiced anxieties similar to mine. But their faces lit up over the course of the evening as, one by one, others in the group echoed their fears.

It was freeing to share our worries out in the open and find out that others struggled with the same things. More than once someone said, "I can't believe you thought that too. I was sure it was only me."

It can also help to clock those times when fear seems to take hold. Some of us experience an increase of unexplained anxiety when our hormones rise or fall. We may not realize that a fear is hormonally related when we're in the middle of it; but if we look back later, we can see the pattern. Then we know to be more on guard at certain times of the month.

But the best antidote for fear is not something *we do* as much as it is something *God has done*. I have always been drawn to the verse, "There is no fear in love. But perfect love drives out fear" (1 John 4:18). Whenever fears rise up, we need to stop whatever we're doing and dip our souls in the truth of that scripture. I find that as I do this, I remember all over again the rock-solid base on which my true security rests. And as I latch on in a fresh way to the understanding of how extravagantly I am and always will be loved by my heavenly Father, I am reassured that *all is well*— because I have this perfect love living in me.

It's so calming to stop and sit once again under the shadow of the Rock that cannot be shaken! Only in that place can I see my fears for what they are: puny, all-mouth emotional bullies. Their strength is nothing compared to the bulging muscles of Jesus—the Older Brother who always comes to pick me up, dust me off, and see that I get safely home.

He will have no fear of bad news; his heart is steadfast, trusting in the LORD. (Ps. 112:7)

👀 In the Chat Room

Shirley, 40: "*My biggest fears are about things like totally losing my memory, female organs dropping, not being attractive enough to keep my husband's interest. I don't want to be old and feeble and too weak to pick things up.*"

Lauren, 44: "*I have a fear of getting cancer or heart disease. I also have a fear of flying or going places unprepared. I'm afraid I'll get to the point that I won't want to go somewhere if it's an unfamiliar place.*"

Lisa, 47: "*Because I'm divorced and not getting any younger, I worry about being single indefinitely and being alone. I actually enjoy my aloneness right now, because I don't have anyone to answer to. I'm very independent, and I like that. But I don't think I want to stay in this place the rest of my life. I worry that the older I get, the less attractive I'll be to someone.*"

Shirlee, 51: "*My biggest fears are of sickness and death. But I've also scared myself a couple of times when I was driving and didn't know where I was, or worse, when I couldn't remember the 'control/alt/delete' procedure on the computer, which is something I do twenty-five times a day.*"

Joann, 59: "*I frequently can't find my words, which used to come easily. All that learning, and sometimes I speak like a second-grader!*"

Suzie, 53: "*My husband and I were on our way to play golf, and I had my tennis shoes on. I was supposed to change into my golf shoes in the car, but by the time we got to the golf course, I had taken my tennis shoes off and put them right back on again. Another time I showed up for church thirty minutes early—the same church I've been going to at the same time for four years. And the other day, I put the milk in the cupboard. I swing from being confident to feeling totally overwhelmed.*"

Martha, 49: "*My intimacy with Jesus sustains me when the bittersweet struggles of life press in on me. It reminds me that this life is not all there is. If I thought this was it, then I would be fearful and depressed. But I see the Bible saying that our older years will be fruitful, and the prospect of eternity with Christ gives us hope.*"

10

[When I can't sleep] I watch the late-night movies on the all-Spanish TV channel, thinking that maybe I can learn a second language.
—Gayle Sand

It's Been a Hard-Dazed Night

2:00 A.M.

For the second time this week I am out in the living room in the middle of the night, plopped on the couch in my robe. Once again the furnace of my affliction has chosen this wee hour to stoke a rousing meltdown, and now I'm fully-flushed-sopping-wet-awake.

I've decided to get up and talk with you because that seems more productive than lying in bed with my mind half open, subject to the jaunts of a rampant imagination that would like nothing more than to put me to work dredging muck from the swamplands of the lives of all of my loved ones. You know how it is—once a mind is awake there is no coaxing it back to sleep, because night brains are forever busy sampling bogus fears acquired from questionable sources.

My husband, David, is also losing the snooze war. Not long ago he could sleep anytime, anywhere, even standing up. Now instead of *Rip Van Winkle*, his bedtime story reads more like *The Princess and the Pea*. Age is part of the problem, but the rest (or lack of it) is due to his sleep mate. Most nights we're like fish flopping in a net. I toss, he turns. He tosses, I turn. Then, all hot and bothered, I flip my pillow to the cool dry side. This goes on and on until one of us gets up.

Hoping for a solution, I started taking an herbal supplement. For a while we were doing well—me doing my part by remembering to take it, the herb doing its part by riding climate-control. Then on vacation I ran out of pills, and, since then everything went up in sweat.

Maybe the pills (or lack thereof) have nothing to do with it, but I need to blame *something* for this new rash of sleep deprivation. I have a hunch I've moved closer to the menopausal force field and more out of the range of plant remedies. Vitamin E doesn't seem to help. The next stop may be hormone replacement. I was hoping to stay off the hard stuff; now I'm not sure I can.

Sleeping in Heavenly Peace

2:30 A.M.

As I think about it, I can see that this whole situation is complicated by the fact that I've grown increasingly fond of sleep—especially the kind of fine quality sleep you get in the World's Most Comfortable Bed, which David and I happen to own.

Everyone who tries our bed agrees it is the most comfortable bed they've ever slept in. This pleases me to no end, because before we bought this bed we had a waterbed (yes, this a rabbit trail; but trust me, it will be worth it) that I was vehemently opposed to getting. But my ultraeager, post-hippie husband knew it would be just the thing for our aching backs, not to mention (*wink, wink*) our love life—which was quite a stretch to picture sitting there sunk in the sloshing plastic at the waterbed store.

I won't trouble you with the whole story, but at the time of this purchase we were also seriously into stockpiling expensive cases of dehydrated food. We had heard we should be prepared in the event of Armageddon or a short-range nuclear disaster. Another genius of the waterbed—said my husband—was that if the end of the world did come and the water supply was compromised, we could keep ourselves alive by siphoning the water from our bed and using it to rehydrate our cheese, rice, and beets. It would be completely safe as long as we were faithful to pour the little blue bottle of chemicals into the rubber plug, which the salesman said was necessary if we didn't want algae building condos under the sheets.

(I told you it'd be worth it.)

The point is, we have finally become real grownups with a luscious, soul-soothing, bona fide mattress—and every once in a while I would like the chance to enjoy it.

What Time Is It in Honolulu?

3:00 A.M

At this moment I am wondering, Are you out there, also wide awake, in High Point, Houston, or Honolulu, with your front-end stuck in the freezer while reading this book? If you were *here*, we could at least entertain each other with Top This Mammogram stories while we snack on calcium-fortified Tums in our sleeveless, superabsorbent, shorty pajamas.

It occurs to me I could pray at a time like this. Not that I'm the type of person who would use prayer as a tranquilizer, but if I were smart I would check to see if God has something he wants to say to me. From what I've read, God likes waking people up when he has a message for them, like the one he gave to Mary: "You are chosen to birth the Messiah." Or to Peter in the middle of a nap: "Hear ye, hear ye, all Hebrews. That previous ban on bacon has now been officially lifted."

I try listening for my own personal message. Nothing comes...

But there is a full moon low in the due west sky, and I can see it through the glass sliding door. When I move it morphs from round to oblong to round again, playing tricks through the screen on the porch. It is a bigger-than-normal moon. In fact it's gigantic, and its brightness casts a weird, eclipselike haze across the backyard.

That is an uncommonly good moon, I think. People should see it. But everyone everywhere is sleeping. They're missing the whole thing! Tonight if you snooze, you lose.

What is it about moons? What is it about *this* moon? Maybe there is a message after all.

Somehow I get the feeling this moon is meant for me— that it has been sent by Someone to keep me company. Maybe it's a lunar "rainbow" proclaiming the promise that the God of All Glory, my God, never changes or sleeps; that he moves and broods through the night like a ready watchman while the earth lies slack and still; that he is neither blind nor idle, even concerning the things that keep a feverish woman up at night.

82

I want to say, "Yes, this is true." But the doubt in me wants a little more proof. I need to know that God is really, acutely involved at the core of my lava-laced midlife.

Of course moons don't talk. But if this one could, I think it would say: "Oh, we see you all right, the Father and I. We see you there on the couch in your waffle-weave robe. We work nights, you know. And every single night for a zillion years to come, the Father will be here sketching a moonscape of me, regardless if anyone sees. He gets a lot of work done when no one is looking."

Good Night, Moon

3:30 A.M.

The moon is gone, and I am back in my room, a cool ninety-eight-point-six. My prince is resting peacefully on his pea. And on the desk beside The World's Most Comfortable Bed, I have scratched a note on the back of a bank statement envelope. It reads: "Tonight you were given a moon-bow."

In the Chat Room

Lisa, 47: *"Restless sleep was a big problem for me. I take natural proges-terone at night, and I sleep better—not perfect, but better. I've had hormone testing several times, and my levels show up in the 'normal' range (what-ever that means)."*

Sue, 53: *"The biggest changes I've seen in myself at midlife are sleepless-ness, wrinkles, dryness, age spots...and getting my feelings hurt more easily. All this bothers me."*

Lauren, 44: *"I take Estroven because I started having night sweats. I've only had them a few times since. I sleep much better now. I'm all about fix-ing the problem."*

Anne, 48: *"I'm not terribly moody, but I do find that I feel anxious at times. That's new for me. Sometimes I lie in bed at night and realize I feel anxious, but I'm not sure why. I do worry sometimes about something happening to my kids, like injury or death."*

The heavens declare the glory of God; the skies proclaim the work of his hands. Day after day they pour forth speech; night after night they display knowledge. (Ps. 19:1–2)

No More Rude Awakenings

If insomnia is a problem for you, you may want to try herbal or hormone supplements. You can also try a few of these slumber inducers:

- Avoid caffeine late in the afternoon and evening.

- Eat heavier meals early in the day and lighter meals in the evening.

- If you must snack at night, try things like turkey, tuna, bananas, or milk. They contain an amino acid called *tryptophan* that can help you relax.

- Avoid vigorous exercise or stimulating TV programs or movies at least one hour before bedtime.

- Try taking a hot shower or a warm bath with Epsom salts. (Magnesium relaxes the muscles.)

- While preparing for bed, listen to soft music and avoid bright lights.

- Drink milk or take calcium supplements near bedtime.

- Keep the bedroom temperature cool during sleep hours.

- Turn in near the same time each night, even on weekends.

- Get out of bed if you can't sleep. Read, stretch, or do relaxation exercises until you start to feel sleepy.

- Pray aloud about any issues that are causing you anxiety, stress, or fear.

Blasts from the Past
Worth Keeping

Sure, there's a lot that's new and different about our lives now. But as I got to thinking about it, I realized there are tons of things we were introduced to in our childhood, teen, and young-adult years that could still come in handy these days.

Here are a few that come to mind:

Skim milk

Park swings

Nap time

Tea parties

Mr. Green Jeans

Hula hoops

Old Maid

Recess

Banana bikes

Slinky's

Sixth period art class

Slumber parties

Library day

Girl Scout cookies

The town of Mayberry

Field trips to the symphony

Gerry and the Pacemakers

Mood rings (Wouldn't it be nice to have more control over mood swings?)

The Twist

I.D. bracelets (for midlife amnesia)

Penny loafers

Hush Puppies

Flip flops

Nineteen-cent hamburgers

Sloppy Joe sweaters

The Sound of Music

Summer vacation

Grandma's house

Swimming at the lake

Tubing down the river

Church picnics

Car trips

Fifty-nine-cent gasoline

Summer camp

Campfire songs

Sadie Hawkins Day

The phrase, "Don't have a cow about it"

Midiskirts (to hide the varicose veins)

Granny dresses and peasant tops (to hide everything else)

Granny glasses (for reading restaurant menus)

Peace symbols (We all need more peace in our lives.)

Clogs

Desert boots (pure comfort for aching feet)

"Turn, Turn, Turn" by the Birds

"You've Got a Friend" by James Taylor

"Little Country Church" by Love Song

Blind dates (At our age, it helps if a husband/date is partly blind.)

Sit-ins (I need to sit a lot more these days, don't you?)

Love-ins (We all need more love in our lives.)

Laugh-In (We need more laughs too.)

"Madge" the Palmolive manicurist

Wilma-and-Betty friendships

Spin-the-bottle (Some midlife couples need a little encouragement.)

Flower power (A few FTD deliveries a year would be nice.)

The Living Bible

PART 3

Midlife Relationships:
Holding On, Letting Go

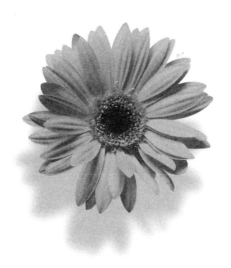

11

The best way to keep your children
home is to make the home
atmosphere pleasant—and let
the air out of the tires.
—Dorothy Parker

Separation Anxiety

These days, there often comes the ever-dawning revelation that my kids are on world-record pace to run off and forget the fabulous life we've shared for the last twenty-some years. Besides sweat-fits, it's the one thing that keeps me up most nights. When I confess this to my husband, he says, "Go to sleep honey. Of course the guys love you. Stop reading into things." But you can't listen to him, because he is always, after all, a father.

If you have a teenager, you probably began to notice suspicious signs of activity around age eleven or twelve, signs only a professionally trained mom knows to look for—certain subtle hints that the young person in question is secretly preparing to enter some sort of Witness Protection Program. These days, for instance, I can leave a message asking our oldest son, who is married and lives across town, to return my call; and it takes days, sometimes weeks, before I hear back from him. A few short years ago this sort of thing would not have been tolerated. We are talking common courtesy here—a character quality that, I happen to know, was heavily stressed in his upbringing.

According to Uncle Sam, our twenty-year-old is still a legal resident of our household, but even the sharpest forensic scientist would have a hard time proving this in a court of law. There are clues that he's been home: a pair of boxers here, a slosh of Gatorade there—no pizza, of course, just the lovely hint of pepperoni dangling in the air.

And now our seventeen-year-old has taken to hugging me funny. I know I should be thrilled that he still hugs me at all. But this new embrace looks a lot like a touch-and-go exercise on an aircraft carrier—next to no contact, no commitment whatsoever. When asked recently about his weak affection, the boy said, "Mom, you're supposed to hug girls different, remember? You told me that." Ah, yes, so I did. A clear case of having my own weapon used against me.

Keeping Our Heads above Water

Understand, I am in no way proposing that we run around doing what certain psychologists and talk-show hosts call "smother-mothering." Smother-mothers are like panicked swimmers who drown anyone who gets near them. These are sad moms who lean on their kids emotionally (instead of the other way around). They control, manipulate, and wreak all sorts of family havoc. Now, I have been accused of wreaking some occasional family havoc myself, but I like my solitude way too much to be a certified smother-mother.

Still, a middle-aged mom needs a safe place to land if she happens to struggle now and then with the process of dismantling the home and family she has spent decades—at great personal expense and exhaustion—to construct. After all, she was told that she must bond with her babies, nurture her little ones, and listen to her teenagers. To a mom, all this means one thing: give them your heart. But once a mom's heart is at full speed, she can't just hit the brakes and put it in park overnight. Not even in a month or two. When a woman has laid down her life and fought for her family spiritually, physically, emotionally, and financially, given the very best years of her life to them, she deserves patience, understanding, and applause—not being told, "Just get over it."

These "just get over it" comments, by the way, usually come from (a) nice but uninformed men, (b) people who didn't like their own mothers, or (c) those who have never had a sweaty-faced child hand them a fistful of flowering weeds and say, "Mommy, I picked these for you."

Where Are the Older Mother Mentors?

At this stage in our lives it would be nice to have some wise, seasoned mentors to show and tell us how it's done. Remember how advice flew in from everywhere when we first got started? Every older woman we knew or passed on the street had a way to deal with feeding, burping, gas, and the fine art of pacification. But I can't seem to remember a single one saying how she handled the process of shutting the door on hands-on motherhood. Even in church circles—where we should be the most sensitive to each other—the subject seems to get glossed over, spoken of as something a mother is meant to endure. Just part of her lot, no complaining, no remorse. *C'est la vie, cherie.*

But it isn't that easy.

When I became a mother, I brought with me into the nursery a good bit of dirty laundry from my own childhood. Raised by a stepmom who gave it her best but rarely connected with us on an emotional level, I grew up feeling unmothered, longing for a mom like the ones all my friends had. So early on I decided: *When I become a mother, I'm going to get it right.*

As my boys were born, I studied them. I catalogued their temperaments, talents, and passions. I celebrated their uniqueness. I read the best child-rearing literature, took classes, listened to tapes, and watched videos. Day in and day out I disciplined, taught, listened to, and hugged them—and then hugged a bit more, always mindful of the lack of affection I'd had as a child.

I wanted to be a fun, creative mom, so we home-schooled, planned field trips, found art classes, and even allowed certain dangerous experiments to be conducted. ("Mom, is it okay if we light a fire in this trash can and throw firecrackers in it?") For who-knows-how-many years, David and I cheered at a zillion baseball, basketball, football, and soccer games. We sat through choir presentations, puppet shows, speeches, and plays. We took a hundred walks and had a thousand talks on everything from God to girls.

I gave the guys my all.

Now, just when they've reached the most delightful stage yet, the party is ending, and I don't want to go home. It's as if the bandleader from one of those old black-and-white movies is standing on the platform and saying, "Folks, all good things must come to an end. This will be the last dance of the evening. Thank you so much for coming."

Where it happened, I'm not sure; but somewhere along the way, my sons got a funny, distracted look in their eyes, as if they had glimpsed the land of Narnia and could no longer bear to play in the wardrobe. Suddenly, Mom—as much as they loved her—was not all-knowing or all-needed. More and more she looked like all those other women in the world.

From Roots to Wings

When the TV miniseries *Roots* first aired, I was in junior high. For some reason, of all those powerful episodes, the scene that has always stuck with me is near the beginning, when the young African boy, Kunta Kinte, gets "manhood lessons."

As the story goes, the tribal fathers appear one day to take Kunta Kinte and several of the other village boys out to a place where they will have to pass a series of mental and physical tests that will graduate them into manhood. Before Kunta Kinte leaves, his mother tells him that when he returns, he will no longer be allowed to live with her. For a moment the boy cries, reluctant to go.

When he eventually returns, something has changed. As he walks past his mother's hut, she eagerly reaches to greet him; but Kunta Kinte stiffens and pretends to ignore her. When she persists, he sternly brushes her off and assigns her a new, lowered status. He refers to her as "woman." Even now I see the pained look on the mother's face as she battles a mixture of pride and betrayal.

Jesus called his mother "woman." In that case, he spoke the words out of kindness for her. Still, the young woman who had carried him and raised him for greatness eventually was left standing at the cross with a mother's shredded heart. This was what she had signed on for, was it not? The whole thing had been in her contract. But now, how to follow through?

I'd like to ask Mary how she was able to shed the authority she once carried. Where did she drop her identity? After decades of tending and loving, how did she hover so near to Jesus, without clutching, right up until the day he died?

All I can guess is she must have gone wading in grace.

I understand grace to be that mystic intangible that walks us through pain to the Peace Room where God lives—if we'll agree to go. Grace is what I need to be bathed in every day in this season of my life. Because even though no one is dying, sometimes it sure feels like it.

When I'm lying in bed at night with that left-behind feeling, David is always good to pat me and say, "Just go on to sleep, honey. This is all part of a bigger plan. Our boys need space for manhood training, you know."

But you can't listen to him—especially now that he's got that funny gleam in his eye, which translated means: "Yahoo! See ya later, boys. Been great having ya. But after twenty-five years of sharing your mama, she's finally all mine again."

In the Chat Room

Mary Lou, 51: *"As a parent, I'm closer to my kids now that they're young adults. It's so great to sit back and enjoy the fruit of all your hard work in raising them. I find I'm doing more listening and not so much lecturing. But not having them at home to create all that excitement and enthusiasm leaves a void."*

Martha, 49: *"The biggest challenge of midlife for me is defining myself. I have always defined myself by my relationships. But age is causing those* relationships to change, so I'm constantly in the process of finding my place."

Shirlee, 51: "I'm trying to listen more to my kids, empower them, not tell them what to do. On Christmas Eve I let my son off the hook so he could be with his fiancée's parents. There was too much pressure on him, and it felt great to free him from my expectations."

Susan, 49: "I get sad and miss my daughter a lot now that she's away at school. I'm working on relinquishing control and relating to all three of my kids adult to adult."

Ginny, 42: "I wish women could start having babies around forty. I feel much more relaxed and at peace with my parenting now."

All my longings lie open before you, O Lord; my sighing is not hidden from you. (Ps. 38:9)

Getting a Grip on Your Empty Nest

Having trouble getting a handle on midlife separation anxiety? Here are two ideas that can help:

Idea #1

Ask a number of older, godly women to share their insights with you about parenting adult children. Ask questions such as:

- How hard was the transition out of hands-on motherhood for you?

- What would you change about the transition?

- What mistakes did you make? What things are you glad you did?

- How were holidays and birthdays different for you after the kids left home?

- What did you find to put in that empty place left behind in your heart?

- Is there such a thing as too much contact with an adult child? If so, what does "too much" look like?

- How did your relationship with Christ sustain you through the hardest parts of the transition from "parent" to "friend"?

Idea #2

Start a Fresh Empty Nesters group. Invite other moms who are facing the same parenting issues you are and facilitate discussion on questions such as:

- What are your greatest fears now that your children have grown up and/or left home?

- What makes you most sad? What are the "upsides"?

- What mistakes have you seen other moms make with kids who've left home?

- Are you finding ways to be an encouragement to your grown children without getting overinvolved in their lives?

- How often do you talk with your children? What seems reasonable?

- Are you spending your time differently now that the kids are grown and/or gone? If so, how?

- Do you have responsibility for your grown children's financial needs, school tuition, car payments, insurance bills, etc.? How do you handle that?

Consider inviting a few older women to tell about their experiences. Share scriptures and draw out more discussion with verses such as these:

- "My grace is sufficient for you, for my power is made perfect in weakness." (2 Cor. 12:9)

- "Even to your old age and gray hairs I am he, I am he who will sustain you. I have made you and I will carry you; I will sustain you and I will rescue you." (Isa. 46:4)

- "Let the peace of Christ rule in your hearts, since as members of one body you were called to peace. And be thankful." (Col. 3:15)

End the evening in a time of prayer for each mom's unique situation. (If the group is large, divide the women two-by-two and ask them to pray for each other.) Consider meeting on a regular basis for ongoing encouragement and support through this challenging season.

12

A son is a son till he takes a wife,
but a daughter's a daughter
all of her life.
—Unknown

Support for Mothers of Males

Based on the way things are heading at my house, all I can say is: If you've been blessed with a daughter, give thanks! Even if you don't care for the guy she's dating or the way she colors her hair, even if (for the moment) you are not on the best of terms, the fact that you have a daughter is significant cause for rejoicing. Why? Because stats from as far back as the Stone Age show that most of the world's daughters live closer to, keep in better contact with, and pay more attention to their middle-aged moms than sons do.

Not that I, the mother of zero daughters, am jealous. But sometime, when he has a minute, I would like to ask God what he had in mind when he shuffled the deck of humanity and dealt my sisters three queens each while slipping me three jacks. Before my family reached its current stage, I was blissfully happy with my lot. Believe me, I love my boys. But the older they get, the more I notice a discrepancy between the sexes.

The Glory of Girls

For instance, I have noticed that a daughter has a way of remembering her mom's favorite color. She remembers her mom's ring size, shoe size, and blouse size (which she knows is not the same as her mom's pants size, but she'll never tell). A daughter is good about calling to find out things like what the doctor said or how the diet's going or to pass on the recipe for Whipped Tofu Fondue she saw on morning TV. She knows the movies her mom has seen and the books her mom has read, and she asks about them. A daughter even knows the day, month, and year her mother was born.

Now your average son (Lord bless him), if asked to recount just one of the above items about you, would likely keel over from a brain freeze. But let GuyTalkRadio throw out a trivia question like, "On lap ninety-one of the Daytona 500, what driver was disqualified for unsportsmanlike conduct the same year Emmett Smith ran for more yards than the combined scores of all the NHL hockey teams in 1977, 1987, and 1997?" and you know full well your son would be the first caller to blurt out to all of Radio Land, "It's Richard Petty's crazy cousin, Hank."

Meanwhile, not only does your average daughter have all of your preferences catalogued—especially after she moves out— she wants to do things with you, such as meeting for lunch at Aunt Pitty Pat's Porch or Victoria's Tea Room and Gardens. In fact, the lunch is likely to be her idea, and she may even bring some kind of gift—maybe a sterling silver pie server, because when she saw it, it reminded her of the times the two of you baked pies together when she was little. Of course this remembrance makes you all watery-eyed, which automatically sets off a similar reaction in her, and something female within her causes her to reach over and squeeze your arm. And for a second or two you sit there all aglow.

Now, your average son would not come within ten football fields of Aunt Pitty Pat's. This is because most boys are born with a-*china*-phobia, which seriously hampers their ability to withstand chitchat, eat from Wedgwood plates, or sit for long periods of time in miniature chairs that have claws where there should be feet.

Boys Know Their Disasters

The news about boys is not entirely grim, however. Sons—especially grown ones—are great to have around in the event of an emergency or natural disaster. (Daughters are little help in these cases, unless you can find some practical use for unbridled hysteria.) A son really shines when, for example, you raise the blinds one morning and happen to see that a sinkhole the size of a semitruck has opened up in your backyard. Or when Storm Tracker 9 reports that a Category One hurricane has been spotted two thousand miles off the coast of Africa and you need someone to tape up the windows.

Such situations call for decisive action—which your average son can solidly handle, because he's spent his childhood watching *McGyver*. From this and other detective shows, a son knows to search the perimeter for suspicious signs of intrusion if you say you've heard a strange noise; and when he is satisfied that you, his mother, are safe, he will then take it upon himself—

without being asked—to fully inspect the contents of your refrigerator (but only as a precaution).

Your average daughter may not know what to do with a disaster, but she is a your kindred spirit. She will sit with you and watch the whole *Anne of Green Gables* trilogy without making a single wisecrack. The innate homing device she was born with keeps her heart always tracking *mom*ward, even when she gets married and moves to Alabama.

Which reminds me of one of the most famous verses in all the Bible, Genesis 2:24: "For this reason a man will leave his father and mother and be united to his wife." Notice it does not say, "For this reason a *woman* will leave her father and mother." Wonder why?

Support Your Local MOMM

Okay, life is not fair. We get what we get, for reasons far beyond our finite comprehension. I understand this. But effective immediately, I am naming myself president of a new global organization called Mothers of Missing Males (MOMM), dedicated to the plight of millions of mothers who will be neglected by their adult sons sometime in the next ten to twenty years. All proceeds will go to developing the first ever "Big Daughters" program, which will encourage and enlist caring young women (regardless of their size) to adopt a MOMM.

The organization will also disseminate the following information so that mothers of daughters know what they can do to help alleviate the suffering of mothers with sons:

- Be sensitive to the depression most mothers of sons face, particularly those mothers in the thick of midlife. Until now we all have been pretty much on pace: same nap times, same field trips, same prom nights, etc. But after graduation it quickly becomes every mom for herself.

- Start MOMM support groups. Invite lonely, left-out moms to your home for in-depth sharing. Moms who seem to have obsessive habits—like filing Missing Persons Reports or tacking photos of their son(s) to random streetlights and telephone poles—are good candidates for this group.

- Share the wealth of your own daughter with a less fortunate mom. When you and your daughter go places like the craft store or the ballet, invite a daughterless mother to tag along. Ask questions about her boy(s). Encourage her to talk about the time her son jumped off the roof and broke his leg or built explosives using lint from the dryer.

- Proudly wear your "I love MOMM" pin and display your MOMM bumper sticker in a prominent location on your car. If seeing one of these reminds even one boy to call his mom or stop by for dinner, it will be well worth poking a hole in your blouse or gunking up your bumper.

No Mistake about the Joy They Make

By now I suppose there's a slight chance you have mistakenly assumed that I am ungrateful for the three highly intelligent, immensely creative, ruggedly handsome young men I have had the privilege of bringing into this world at a measly sacrifice to my C-sectioned, stretch-marked, spider-veined body—those same boys I breastfed, potty trained, home schooled, and cooked, sewed, and vacuumed for. The ones I prayed for, planned parties for, wrestled with, and cried over.

The fun-loving fellows with whom I played patty-cake, peek-a-boo, trucks, monsters, I spy, dress up, hide and go seek, capture the flag, Simon says, red light/green light, Twister, Monopoly, football, baseball, basketball, tennis, bowling, billiards, race cars, skateboard, checkers, cards, and air hockey.

The young men I worked night and day to support, encourage, peptalk, praise, and yell, stomp, clap, and cheer my guts out for.

The unforgettable guys I strolled, bicycled, wagon-rode, grocery carted, merry-go-rounded, swung, burped, cherished, spoiled, pampered, took zillions of pictures of, videotaped, and carted in my body, under my heart, on my back, on my hip, and in my arms.

The precious, priceless boys I kissed and patted and bear-hugged and squeezed and tickled and snuggled and stroked more times per day than the law allows.

Those special ones I tucked in, woke up, bathed, rocked, sang to, smiled at, longed for, and never, ever got tired of staring at or being with.

If previously I gave you the impression that I am in any way sorry for the more than twenty-five years I have invested my body, soul, mind, and spirit into those boys—oh, no. It's the opposite. They have been my highest joy.

Taking One for the Team

The tough part, the part I'm wrestling with, is that they are just about grown and gone, and this is one mom who has never been anything but a player. It's hard being told to sit on the bench now. It's hard to hear, "You stay here while we go play somewhere else." I love being part of my sons' lives. They make me laugh—and keep me young. Besides, why break up a good team?

I know. This is the way families go. But I don't much like it. Of course I will get to see them from time to time. And every now and then they just might let me back in the game to bunt or pinch-hit. Maybe. We'll have to see. You know how boys are.

In the Chat Room

Anne, 48: *"I like parenting at this stage. The kids are more fun. I enjoy and appreciate the fact that I won't have them around much longer. I've tried to pull away and not get as involved in their lives. I'm trying to encourage them to make more decisions on their own."*

Lisa, 47: *"As a parent I'm definitely not as strict as I was. I let my son get away with a lot more than his older sisters ever did at the same age."*

Cathy, 42: *"My kids are even more fun now that we can have adult conversations. But the pulling away of my son is sometimes painful."*

Martha, 49: *"My daughters and I relate more as friends now. We love doing things together. It's such a blessing that they want me to go places and do things with them. But it can be a bit confusing trying to figure out when to step in and when to stay out of their lives. From nursery through college, I've always been very involved with my daughters' activities. It's a stretch for a 'fix everything' mom to let them become adults."*

I will lead the blind by ways they have not known, along unfamiliar paths I will guide them; I will turn the darkness into light before them and make the rough places smooth. These are the things I will do; I will not forsake them. (Isa. 42:16)

13

My mother's death was the dividing line between seeing the world in black and white and in Technicolor....I was never again going to be able to see life as anything but a great gift.

—Anna Quindlen

What's Really Eating the Sandwich Generation?

Among the many unsettling outgrowths of middle age is the feeling you sometimes get that all the important people in your life are sneaking off to a luscious, fun spot somewhere, and you are not invited. I felt that way at age nine, when my parents left my sisters and me at home with our grandmother so they could buy straw hats and ride around the Bahamas on motor scooters. Babies know this feeling, too, from all the times their mothers bribe them to sleep, then sneak out of their rooms, praying like crazy.

What causes this sensation in midlife is the growing evidence of a mass exodus of biblical proportions taking place at two significant relational poles: Our kids exit stage left, while our parents exit stage right.

All Out of Bread

If you're like me, you're probably getting a bit weary of being referred to as the Sandwich Generation. I think people call us this because (a) we find ourselves smack in the middle of—and stretched beyond all recognition by—the tension of caring for our kids on the one hand and our parents on the other; and (b) as children we were forced to consume more Skippy peanut butter than any other generation in world history.

What really happens is that, after our kids leave home (provided they don't move back), we are left with only the bottom half of our sandwich, at which point we become the Open-Faced Sandwich Generation. Then, when our parents pass to the other side, we turn into the Diet Plate Generation, and our team fight song becomes that great golden oldie: "The cheese stands alone, the cheese stands alone, hi-ho-the-dairy-o, the cheese stands alone." No one really advertises that part.

Perhaps you're thinking that all this talk makes me sound suspiciously like someone with abandonment issues. While I do confess expertise in that particular arena, I believe feelings are meant to be felt—as we'll discuss in a later chapter. It's no crime to have intense feelings—especially feelings of abandonment, because, after all, you never asked for these feelings in the first place; and besides, you're the *leave-ee*, not the *leave-er*.

Anyway, any number of extra-raw parent-child/child-parent emotions are bound to surface in middle age, and the healthiest way I know to deal with the little monsters (the emotions, not the children) is to herd them all out into the daylight, where we can get a good look at them.

Of course, we (okay, *I*) have already done some serious moaning in previous chapters about the void left by our vanishing offspring. We won't rehash all that here. Instead, I want to devote the rest of this chapter to the shocking, slap-in-the-face, nonconsideration of our feelings that happens when our parents (of all people) permanently vacate the premises. The truth is, as we've gotten older, our parents have gotten *even older* than the "old" we used to think they were when we thought we knew everything. I don't have to tell you that this can be one of the scariest revelations in life. Which is why I want to walk you through what's ahead.

If you have already experienced the pain of losing your mom or dad, you will probably identify with parts of my story. If both your parents are alive (whether they're healthy or not), be thankful. Cherish them. Buy them lots of gifts and denture adhesive. And store this chapter away—for another day.

She Just Couldn't Say No

In my case, cigarettes were to blame.

Mom was raised in the Tobacco Capital of the Universe at a time when one puff on a Marlboro could pretty much guarantee you a date with Cary Grant. Multiply that scenario by forty-five years, combine it with diabetes, and you get no-turning-back-now heart damage, not to mention kamikaze blood pressure and a five-needle-a-day insulin habit. But even through all that, Mom refused to divorce her beloved cigarettes. So about three years ago, her body had no choice but to give her a heart attack.

After this attack came five-bypass surgery, pacemaker/defibrillator implants, and, for me, the heart-halting realization that our mom was on borrowed time. Thank God for borrowed time! The best thing about it is that you get to say and do things you wouldn't have the guts to say and do if the "big eraser" (as Anne Lamott calls it) were to suddenly swoop down without warning.

Everybody's Got Issues

As with most families, ours had a few cracks in the plaster. Mom was actually our stepmother. When our Dad died very young, she was left to raise my sisters and me, alone, full time. And for reasons it would take a whole other book to explain, through our years together there came several seasons of serious estrangement in our relationship, which created some weird, disabling gaps in our emotional connectedness to her.

By the time Mom got sick, those days were long forgiven. But despite an unbroken roll of good years together, every now and then those old scars got scratched open, and I'm sorry to say we didn't always ask, "What would Jesus do?" when it came to Mom's neediness.

But we were family—the only family Mom had left. (Well, she did have one cousin in Virginia and a nephew she hadn't spoken to in twenty-some years.) So it was the duty of my sisters and me to see that Mom was taken care of. To be blushingly honest, we sometimes resented having to interrupt the *important* things we were doing to drive her to a doctor's appointment. Sometimes we wrestled over whose turn it was to pick up a prescription at the pharmacy, deal with Social Security and Medicare, or sit with Mom in the hospital. (She was there eighteen times in three years.)

Since Mom couldn't work, we took money from our own budgets to help cover hers. Due to various circumstances, however, we didn't always have equal opportunity to share in this coverage—which occasionally caused a little tension in the sisterhood.

A Not-So-Welcome First

Then, one evening, while David and I were out of town on vacation, Mom and a friend sat down to watch *Jeopardy*. Mom had just taken a bite of a cheese sandwich when she looked up at her friend and said, "Did you bring your stethoscope?" After that she slumped over unconscious.

By ten o'clock the next morning, Mom was gone.

Thankfully, David and I were able to get back quickly and be with Mom in her last hours. Her death was the first one I actually witnessed. Before that time I had seen people in coffins, but I had never watched someone die.

Mom's passing wasn't exactly peaceful, like you sometimes see in the movies. She was in a coma, and after they turned off the respirator and pulled the tube from her throat, she began to make frighteningly sudden gasping and rattling sounds. Experts say that people in comas can't hear anything; but just in case doctors don't know everything, I talked to Mom anyway (when I wasn't crying). I stood by the bed stroking her hair and forehead, repeating over and over, "Mama, we're all here…all your girls are here…and God is here…we're sure going to miss you…I love you, Mama." Funny thing, I hadn't called her Mama since childhood.

All of us—my sisters, our husbands, four of the grandkids, and I—held hands around her bed. Through our tears we thanked God for Mom's life, for what she had given us, and especially for the last ten or so years that had wonderfully rewritten what might have been a not-so-happy ending to our story together. Hospital staff kept checking in on her from time to time. They were nice about it, but you could tell that to them, someone's mother dying was something akin to brushing your teeth.

For three hours we thought she would die any minute. We stood there with our eyes fixed on her chest. Finally she sucked one quick gasp, then another, then her shoulders froze mid-breath. They never came back down, the way they do in a normal exhale. She was stuck there, hunched up, eyes closed, and mouth locked half-open. It was as if she had been poked in the ribs—as if someone had asked her, "What's going on here?" and she had answered, "Beats me." In seconds her skin went from pink to yellowish gray to gray. We could actually see this happening. Finally I leaned over, my face in her hair, and wept hard into the pillow.

To think that only the day before, I had been sitting under a beach umbrella, lamenting to myself that our vacation was almost over.

Good-bye Children, Hello Heaven

Mom's funeral was triumphant. Prior to the service, her casket was open. I just couldn't do the cremation thing (though I respect those who might choose that route). Mom was in the black cocktail dress she wore for our oldest son's wedding, with a string of faux pearls we found in her room and some earrings we bought her one Christmas. I asked my daughter-in-law, Becca, who is from Hawaii, to make a lei of pink carnations, which we also placed around Mom's neck. (For future reference: At the funeral home, the guy in charge asked me, "Did you bring Mrs. Chandler any undergarments?" Well, no. It never occurred to me that the deceased might need undergarments.)

Lying there, Mom did not look like herself. But it was good to have at least a fair representation—especially for her friends who wanted to say good-bye. Before her casket was closed, many of us took letters we had written to her and tucked them inside. That was tough, closing the casket. But then someone played the Doxology, and we all stood up and sang. Singing is so good for grief, even though it's the last thing you feel like doing.

Next, one of our staff pastors told some funny stories he knew about Mom and invited others to come forward and share what she had meant to them. Many did, and their words were priceless. In a lovingly honest way, David recounted the story of Mom's life, mingling it with Scripture as he described the herky-jerky transformation we'd made as a family over time. He talked in particular about the changes God had brought about in Mom.

Afterward, each sister got up and shared something. When it came my turn, I read a copy of the letter I'd put in the casket:

Dear sweet, precious Mom:

I can't believe we are doing this today. I can't believe this is real. My heart aches and grieves at the thought that you have left us forever.

I am thankful for the last three years—even as hard as they have sometimes been—because they have given us a little time to begin thinking toward this day...this hour. I am so thankful we did have some warning and could say many things to each other. But even though we knew the possibility of you dying was ever-increasing, I am still not prepared to live my life with you absent. I'm not sure how I will do it. You have been the strongest, longest force in my life. For forty years we have shared quite the journey, haven't we?

I will miss seeing you tear up as we all hold hands around the table at Thanksgiving to pray and share our thankfulness. I will sorely miss your cornbread and mashed potatoes.

I will miss your faithful presence at church each week, and I know it will take a long time before I will remember not to look for you there.

I will miss you at birthdays and those times when just the girls get together. I will miss how we laughed to the point of tears (and other unmentionables) just remembering some of the crazy things that happened when we all lived under one roof.

I will oh-so-much miss that look on your face you'd get when you hugged our boys and bragged about how wonderful they all are. I will miss the way they laughed at you when you didn't even know you were funny.

I will miss the way you delighted in me.

I will miss the shy way you asked us to pray for you when you were sick or afraid.

I will miss the times you talked about Daddy. And I am curious to know if you have run into him yet.

What a joy it has been to watch you grow and change these last many years. From now on, for the rest of my life, I know I will have the ache of missing your constant, gentle presence somewhere near me. Thank you for the many years and many ways you tried to dedicate your life to my family and me...even after all we've been through.

Mama, how different all this is from what I thought it would be. I hurt at a much deeper place than I have known. It will take God to hold me up when these waves of grief hit me out of nowhere.

Please, please know how treasured you have been and forever will be. And just one more time, I'd like you to hear from me that I love you so very, very much.

At the end of the funeral we showed a great video of Mom's life, set to LeAnn Rimes's song "Please Remember." (Mom was a serious country fan.) Edited by Joseph, our seventeen-year-old, the video included the only footage we had of Mom and Daddy together. They were in their twenties, doing what Dad used to call "horsing around" in a swimming pool. How sweet and achy-sad it was to see them there on the screen, to know they were both gone now. I pretty much lost it at that point.

Then, by the strength of her three grandsons and three sons-in-law, Mom was carried on to her grave.

A Funny Thing Happened on the Way to the Funeral

Did I mention that the night before the funeral, Becca and I, along with my sisters and their six daughters, worked on a flower arrangement to put on top of Mom's casket? We chose fifty-plus long stemmed, pink roses, plus some carnations and a few other flowers I liked the looks of. Anyone can buy florist-arranged flowers; what I wanted was for all of us to put our hearts and hands into honoring Mom in a personal, original way. I figured I knew enough about flower arranging to pass for knowledgeable. And besides, I have always been in favor of doing something other than what most people do (as long as it doesn't get you in trouble).

Understand, we had no backup plan. Since the funeral was early the next morning, there would be no way to get a florist to rescue us if our attempt failed.

That evening was a great bonding time. The ten of us worked on the arrangement, told "Mammaw stories," and laughed at silly things—which we encouraged each other to do whenever we felt like it, no crime or disrespect to the dead. (Mom would have insisted we laugh.) When we finished, our floral masterpiece could have passed for something out of an FTD catalogue—no exaggeration. We all agreed that the sight of it would have set Mom off like fireworks. She was like a child that way.

On its way to the church the next morning, however, jostled as it was in the back of my brother-in-law's van, our great work of art did a serious parting-of-the-Red-Sea imitation. It split right down the middle, flowers flopping every which way. At that point, one sister went berserk. We couldn't possibly have flowers so…unprofessional! Casket flowers are supposed to be a focal point. Not to mention, we had bragged to the entire world (via the funeral bulletin) that we, Mom's daughters and granddaughters, were responsible for the beauty set before them.

I tried to calm everyone down (that's pretty much been my assignment since the start of the space program) and propped up the flowers as best I could. Somehow they held together through the service—which is all we had asked them to do in the first place. Then, as everyone gathered at the graveside and the funeral home guy (with his most ceremonious *plop*) sat our now-withered labor of love on top of the casket one last time, the whole arrangement keeled over—just disintegrated right in front of everyone—sending roses prematurely down into the open vault.

What could we do, sitting there on the front row, staring at this sorry-excuse-for-nothing at the final earthly tribute to our mother? Nothing you *can* do but laugh. You know, the kind of laugh that comes after crying? Thankfully, only our closest friends and family were there to see the catastrophe. They laughed, too, but theirs was more of a nervous, somebody-please-do-something-this-is-terrible kind of laugh.

Honestly, Mom would have wet her pants.

Afterthoughts

It rained that night. As I sat on the porch and watched the water drip off the roof, I felt a new, vacant sadness. And I thought, *Here we are, all dry and alive, while our mom lies under the dirt out in the rain. We are just going to leave her out there—in the rain—and no one is going to do anything about it, because this is the way it's supposed to go when someone dies. Within hours of burying a person who had been moving around on the earth for sixty-five years, you're not supposed to worry or think thoughts about them smothered underground. How strange is that?*

I didn't sleep well that night.

A few days later, I wrote an e-mail to a friend and told her the whole story. Through that process I realized there were a number of things I was grateful for:

- I was glad Mom was not alone when she had her stroke.

- I was glad she never knew that on top of *everything else* that was wrong with her, she also had a brain tumor.

- I was glad she didn't have to live in a paralyzed state, as some stroke victims do (although I would have been more than happy to take her in any condition).

- I was glad I took her to the airport the day the kids left on their mission trip. Mom wanted to be there—*had* to be there, she said—to see the grandkids off. Something in me said, "Take her." It was her last good-bye to them.

- I was glad I told Mom I loved her before David and I left for our vacation. After church the Sunday before, I gave her a quick kiss and said, "Keep an eye on the boys for me while I'm gone. I love you." I'm pretty sure I said that last part. It was our last exchange. (Strange how you never realize the significance of these moments at the time. You just go on about your plans as if we will all be here forever.)

- I was glad we were able to get home quickly and be with Mom when she slipped into heaven. She so much would have wanted that.

- I was glad she had the best life we knew how to give her. And I was glad that what we had to give her was what she really needed most.

- Most of all, I was glad for the astounding love and grace of God that found a way to carve a sweet, sensitive grandma out of a once sad and bitter stepmom.

Mom did sneak off to a luscious fun spot—a place full of more delight than I can comprehend. But she didn't go anywhere that I'm not invited to follow. In fact, I've already sent my RSVP. It's just the date that's still a little fuzzy.

In the Chat Room

Martha, 49: *"My father, who has always been the healthiest parent, just had open-heart surgery. Things are beginning to transition as I watch my parents needing more help. Right now we're discussing the possibility of them uprooting their home and moving closer so I can better help them. This would be a big deal, but it will most likely be necessary."*

Lisa, 47: *"I have a very loving relationship with my parents. But it's strained at times because of their health problems, and we live a great distance apart."*

Anne, 48: *"I feel like I've become the parent and my mother the child. Both my brothers live in other countries, so I'm it for my mom. That can be suffocating at times. She has not been well, and recently we moved her into an apartment. I lost my dad three years ago, and I'm amazed how well I handled it, even though we were very close. I think it's because I knew he was ready and thought he'd had a wonderful life."*

Wanda, 51: *"It was a blessing to be with my mom when she died. We took care of her at home. I was surprised at the grief I felt. Just knowing you don't have a mom here on earth anymore is sad. But my father is active, and we have a good relationship."*

Jackie, 46: *"My mother was sick for a long time, and it was kind of a relief to not have to worry about her anymore. I miss her. For two years after she died, I had dreams about her. My dad is in a care home in another city. My role with him now is mostly just to keep in touch and visit from time to time."*

Cathy, 42: *"I took care of my mother and both my in-laws before they died. It was hard, but I'm glad I did it. I have a lot of good memories, and I knew them all even better for it. But I still miss my mother. I would love to ask her questions about midlife and how I was as a teenager, now that I have teens of my own."*

June, 59: *"I'm becoming the primary caregiver as my parents become more dependent in their eighties. I'm actually excited at the prospect of having them around, especially since they are not believers. I get to be Jesus to them!"*

Lauren, 44: *"I still miss my mom a lot. Sometimes there's a split second when I think she's still here and start to pick up the phone to call her."*

Now may the Lord of peace himself give you peace at all times and in every way. (2 Thess. 3:16)

Jesus, I Need Your Prayers Today

Dear Jesus,

The further I get in this unique time in my life, the more I see what a radical passage it is. I was hoping that some of the rumors weren't true—that the paradigm shift wasn't as great as, say, first-time parenthood or moving to a Third World country. But this is like a foreign country sometimes—and you know from my high-school French class that I'm not great with languages. And while, now and then, I like road trips, I don't crave travel that much.

So that's why I need your prayers today.

I've read the prayers you prayed in Jerusalem, and since you're the same yesterday, today, and forever, I have an idea about the kind of prayers you are praying right now. It seems a constant theme of yours was, "Your will be done, Father…Your kingdom come, on earth—right here—as in heaven…Let this cup pass from me; but if it cannot, then your will be done, not mine." And knowing the mission you were given, I can see why you would place a premium on not getting tangled up in your own aspirations and preferences. Still, for the record, if I could pass up this cup…If I could skip the requirement to taste it, or at least certain bitter parts, that would be good…If there's anything you can do….

So, you see, I need you to pray for me. You knew the conflicting emotions of hosting a farewell dinner, taking up your cross, redirecting your mother's love from yourself to someone else. There was pain—no, torture—in walking all of that out, and my situation is hardly a gnat's eye compared to it. But I can relate in a small way to the conflict, and to the call of the Bigger Picture. Pray that I become a "yes woman." Pray for growing cooperation on my part with every directive passed down from the Home Office. And pray that I can find creative ways to be strengthened by the changes I'm going through rather than paralyzed by them.

I need you to pray for me, Jesus, because on my own I have never been a super great pray-er, as you well know. Cover me with your shield, because the enemy is licking his chops. I don't want to give him my business. Pray that I won't accept an alternate plan—only the one you have set before me.

Today I'm in need of a grace lift—a renewed state of being— beyond anything I can do in my own power to alter my countenance and lift up my head. Pour out your oil of gladness. Speak to my soul; share with me the secrets you used when you walked up your hill. Since you "always live to intercede," I make this appeal.

I know you are praying today, so I ask for new eyes—not to read better but to rest better, both in you and in your path for my life. I ask that you flood the eyes of my soul with light, the kind that wipes away the shadows. I need light—your Light—to expose all those precious gems you say you have placed along my way, to show me the good you're about in this season. Because I know you are all about good.

Jesus, I need your prayers today. I need to know that you see me here in all my female humanity; that you're aware of all these changes along the road; that you are counting the tolls and sending down strength and courage and power to allow me to pass through them. I need to feel your nearness. I have exceeded my weight limit, and I am unable to fly on my own. Will you lift this burden as you promised you would, if I would just lean into you?

Well, here it is, Lord, the whole lot of it. My entire life, such as it is at the moment. I know you will take it and make something beautiful. You always do.

Caron

14

You don't need to be afraid of change. You don't have to worry about what's been taken away. Just look to see what's been added.
—Jackie Greer

Did Somebody Say the G-Word?

I never said we don't need grandmothers. I am enormously grateful for my own grandmothers—all three—who were good to send vitamins, toothbrushes, and self-addressed, stamped envelopes. They taught me to sew and crochet, and even how to drive. I think everyone should have a sweet, spoil-you-rotten-grandmother (or at least someone in the neighborhood who can serve as a secondhand, stand-in grandma if the real one lives elsewhere). Grandmothers are great.

I'm just not ready to be one.

Normally an admission like this would be no big deal. But the situation has become time-sensitive: My oldest son, Joshua, and his sweet bride, Becca, have gone behind my back and, in three months, will make me a grandmother—whether I'm ready or not.

From general observation I gather my attitude is a freak of female nature, because most of the women I talk to are ecstatic at the prospect of grandchildren. My sister, who is three years younger than me, can hardly wait for the occasion. Some of my friends talk about it like dieters craving chocolate.

So what's the matter with me? I have nothing against grandchildren. I love children. It's just that grandkids have a corresponding grandma, and that's the part that's tripping me up.

The Problem with Grandma

I feel too young to be a grandmother. I realize that, technically, age has nothing to do with it. Theoretically, a thirty-year-old could be a grandmother. It's just that about 75 percent of the grandmothers I know look the part. From earliest memory all of my grandmas carried themselves like a grandmother should (with the exception of one who, well into her eighties, kept us delighted with her ever-trendy wardrobe). But even when they were young, my grandmas seemed old to me. That's why, at this barely midstage of life, I find it hard to get up the heart to go there.

You hear folks say that people looked older back then. We're fitter, healthier nowadays. That may be true, but it's still pretty tough to erase those images of blue lacquered hair, quilting bees, and rocking chairs when you grew up glued to the antics of the cranky little granny on *The Beverly Hillbillies*.

Besides, there are no good "grandmother" names. This probably sounds about as trite as it gets, but if you must be assigned a new post, the least they can do is give you a title that lets you hold up your head. I agree they were headed in the right direction when they started with the word *grand*. But from what I can tell, there have been no stellar improvements in the names assigned to grandmothers in the last eight hundred years. You've still got your basic Gran, Grammy, Granny, Nanny, Nana, Nini, Ma, and Mimi; and for more continental types, Grandmere (French), Grobmutter (German), Nona (Italian), Avo (Portuguese), Abuela (Spanish), Oma (Dutch), and so on. None of these names sound like me.

Someone proposed I wait about a year and let the baby name me himself. I'm not too keen on this technique. They tried it in my daughter-in-law's family, and to this day (absolute true story) they call Rebecca's grandmother "Butt-Tee."

Here's an interesting note. While searching through the Internet one day, I found a site called Grandboomers ("where baby boomers meet the grandchildren"). According to Grandboomers, what to name a new grandparent is the most frequent e-mail question they get. So, see, it's not just me.

Look Who's Driving

On that fateful night last November when Josh and Becca announced they had officially been called up for diaper duty, I knew how I was supposed to react. I knew how everyone wanted me to react. And I knew how I wished I could act. Plenty of women (my own mother-in-law for one) have worldwide reputations for hooting and hollering their heads off at the news of such a blessed event.

But for me, it was as if someone had stuck a vacuum to my lungs. I felt shoved head-first into the Future, even though I was still not quite done with the Present, thank you. Inside there came a chilling, quickening sadness—sick and self-centered as that sounds—a silly, shuddering sadness, because a new era was about to be birthed for me, whether I liked it or not. It felt as if someone wanted to stuff Mom in the rumble seat, when she still had a lot of drive in her.

And so, as these two newly married novices stood on the sidewalk grinning and beaming and waving their ultrasound photo, all David and I could muster after a long, awkward pause was, "Wow, guys...this is...wow."

Grandma: The Role of a Lifetime

One of the things running through my mind at that moment was how much stage a twelve-pound infant can steal. There is nothing (I repeat, nothing) more entertaining than watching your chubby-cheeked offspring do tricks on the living room floor. A baby would mean that all the great times we'd been sharing as a family would center less and less around our kids and us parents and more around the new parents and their bouncing, burping bambino. Conversations would switch from stretching and stimulating discussions to delirious demonstrations of "dada," "bye-bye," and "potty chair."

It hit me that more than all the graduations, weddings, and home-leavings combined, a grandchild would alter the script of our family once and for all. I remembered my own mom's experience and how much a grandchild changed things. The new recruit ended up unhinging her from the lead, care-giving "Mom" role she had always known and cast her from that day forward into the part of "Mammaw." (To her great credit, she never seemed to regret this change. Instead, she smartly stepped up to the plate, and in grand fashion out-performed all her earlier seasons as a mom.)

Standing there that night in all speechlessness, I saw my life slipping past me—sensed it flying right out of my hands, as life is prone to do. For a moment I felt lost and afraid. I couldn't sense God, but my brain knew better than to think this sudden life shift had somehow missed his scope. I've been around long enough to know that this deed, like so many others before, had been done on earth as it was in heaven. Clearly, God was writing me new lines for a new part, and it was my job now to learn and deliver them with all my heart.

What's a Mother to Do?

Since then I've done a lot of thinking about my new, upcoming role. And I've decided that if I'm going to be successful, I've got to lean my weight on the mega-catalogued witness of all those millions of women who've grandma-ed before me. Since they already know the way, I need to study their maps and choose to believe that the ride is just as exhilarating as they say—and that a few months from now I will be every bit as annoyingly grandchild-obsessed as they have ever been.

I also need to apply some of the wisdom I heard years ago from a dear, weathered saint, who told me not to worry about having enough love to go around. While carrying my second child, I became concerned that I couldn't love two children as well as I had loved one. "When the time comes," this wise woman said, "God will not ask you to split your love in half. He will multiply it over and over and over with brand-new batches of love for as many babies as he gives you." I'm suspecting this goes for my children's children too.

And last (but probably most important), I've got to believe that all this passion, vigilance, and commitment I've put into mothering my three sons will somehow, by God's design, make a seamless, binding transfer over to little Gavin Chandler Koa

Loveless—from the very first moment his weepy-eyed grandma picks him up and cradles him softly in her arms.

Did I just say the G-Word?

But the plans of the LORD stand firm forever, the purposes of his heart through all generations. (Ps. 33:11)

◦◦ In the Chat Room

Lisa, 47: *"When I feel good and the grandchildren are behaving, being a grandma is the sweetest thing in the world. I have as much love for them as I do for my very own. But on the other days, I'm so glad I can send them home."*

Jackie, 46: *"I've had lots of trouble with the loss-of-control issues. I worry when my kids are out on the roads at night. Sometimes I just miss putting them down for the night and knowing they're safe. I wonder how my children not needing me anymore will affect me, but I'm looking forward to grandchildren."*

Karen, 65: *"When our grandchildren were born, they were the dearest bundles of joy. How I love those little ones! But I don't give advice to my kids about parenting. I don't have the authority now. I just complain to Grandpa whenever I see them not disciplining their own kids."*

Joann, 59: *"I should be rocking grandbabies...but I'm arguing with teenagers and rocking grandbabies. Oh, but I love, love, love being a grandmother!"*

Books to Rock Grandma's Socks Off

Hugs for Grandma by Chrys Howard (Howard Publishing Company)

Funny, You Don't Look Like a Grandmother by Lois Wyse and Lilla Rogers (Crown Publishing)

When a Child Is Born, So Is a Grandmother by Mary Engelbreit (Andrews McMeel Publishing)

The Nanas and the Papas: A Boomers Guide to Grandparenting by Kathryn Zullo and Allan Zullo (Andrews McMeel Publishing)

Totally Cool Grandparenting by Leslie Linsley (St. Martin's Press)

The Grandmother Book by Betty Southard (Thomas Nelson)

15

When I pictured myself in my fifties—if I ever did—it certainly wasn't as a recess monitor.
—Marcelle Clements

She's Having a Baby... at Forty!

Though the Bible declares, "Like arrows in the hands of a warrior are sons born in one's youth" (Ps. 127:4), it also gives much press to the birth of the late-in-life babies of women such as Sarah, Rachel, Hannah, and Elizabeth. From the Old Testament to the New, these accounts instruct us on faith, trust, and the faithfulness of God to keep his promises.

For many women, today's babies-come-lately teach similar lessons. And whether the reason is midlife remarriage, a surprise pregnancy, a decision to postpone maternity in pursuit of a career, or a delay caused by infertility, the number of women having babies in the prime of life is on the rise.

At any age, having a baby means sacrifice. But when the mother is older than most, the demands on her body, soul, and spirit subtract a unique toll—and also return a unique joy. One woman who knows the gamut of these emotions in a fresh way is my good friend and ministry assistant, Leslie Aziz, who recently shared her account of midlife maternity with me. The next few pages are written in her own words.

Foolish at Forty?

Some years ago I read *Pavilion of Women* by Pearl S. Buck. One of the main characters reaches the age of forty and has a baby—a really bad thing to do, since she's living in China in the early 1900s.

In the way book ideas sometimes shape our own thoughts, I half expected someone like Buck's character to walk up to me during my own pregnancy and point out my foolishness for wanting and conceiving a second baby in my forties. I received, of course, not even a sideways glance. Modern society seems to accept—no, celebrate—women having babies at the onset of middle-agedom.

But that doesn't mean it's easy.

One day during my pregnancy, I walked through my office and noticed a friend sitting in the reception area. When she saw me, she asked how I felt.

"Tired," I answered. "This pregnancy makes me feel really tired."

"You'd be tired anyway," she responded. "You're forty."

She's a little farther into her forties than I am, so even though we both laughed, I knew she spoke from substantial experience—and I secretly shuddered. *Feedings around the clock, doing housework while holding a newborn, not to mention the necessary energy just to give birth—I'm forty, for Pete's sake. I can't do this!* Then Emma Grace poked a tiny foot into my forty-year-old side, and joy disguised as youthful vim helped me pick up my step and hum.

I woke up in labor. The clock said 3:45 A.M., and my contractions were already three minutes apart.

When we got to the delivery room, I happened to glance at my hospital chart. There, written in six-inch letters across both pages, were the words *Advanced Maternal Age.* The notice was surely medi-code for what the delicately perfumed nurses were too polite to say: "This old woman doesn't have the stamina to push out a baby."

As it turned out, I only pushed for forty-five minutes before Emma was born—something to really applaud since I did a VBAC (vaginal birth after cesarean). This was, in fact, the first time my Advanced-Maternal-Age body had delivered a baby naturally.

Holding Emma in the gentle moments that followed (even as muffled delivery screams from the room adjacent to mine seeped through the wall), I was awed at the glory of birth and filled with joy to think that such glory should come to me in my new middle-agedness. Her quiet breathing sang lullabies to whatever worries I'd had about missed sleep and foolish choices.

For Such a Time as This

She is beautiful. Really. I'm not just speaking as her mother. A few months before Emma's birth, a friend—not someone especially close, but more than an acquaintance—

told me she couldn't sleep the previous night because of Emma. At first I laughed and said, "I'm sorry she kept you up." Then I looked into my friend's face and realized that something significant had happened to her the night before.

"She's like Esther. I couldn't sleep last night and felt compelled to read Esther. God is telling me she is like Esther, Esther the beautiful queen."

Beauty given for God's purpose and glory! Not one time have I taken Emma somewhere—the grocery store, the pharmacy, 7-Eleven—and at least one stranger hasn't stopped us and said, "What a beautiful baby! What's her name?" Just today, as I pushed my way down the cereal aisle with Emma sitting up in the child's portion of the shopping cart, a woman turned into the same aisle and startled me.

"Oh, my goodness! Isn't she adorable—and so petite! How old is she?"

I told her Emma's age, and the lady cooed, "Well, she is just the sweetest thing!"

Sometimes I press Emma's cheek next to mine, and we look in the giant bathroom mirror. I'm forever surprised at my face. The bags under my eyes practically swallow my eyelids when I smile; there's an entire streak of gray insolently growing on the right side of my part; and an unmistakable jowl line appears regardless of what unnatural angle I hold my head. I hate this part of forty.

Then I move my eyes from me to her, and none of it matters. My face is Emma's joy, her comfort, her door to the world, and indeed—for now—her identity. And in her gaze, I feel God's love. His complete acceptance of me is there, reflected in the unconditional love in her eyes.

Light My Fire

I've read it in magazines and heard it on morning shows, but it's one cliché that's true for me: Women reach their sexual peak in their forties. At forty I've finally attained enough sense to shed the old notion that an ideal body equals romance. And by now I have enough bedroom experience to communicate with my husband, so we know how to light each other's fires. I love this part of forty!

But while I was pregnant and for the couple of months that followed, sex seemed like a vacation memory: I knew it had happened, I remembered it was a great time, but I didn't expect to go there again. For a month after her birth, Emma teetered on the cusp of low weight gain, and her pediatrician told me repeatedly, "Don't let that baby sleep! Wake her up every two to three hours around the clock to nurse." The only fire I felt in those days was the burning under my eyelids.

But she did gain weight. She even fell easily into a 7:30-ish bedtime. Now round-the-clock feedings are the memory. These days I can peek into my seven-year-old's room and see him peacefully tangled in his blankets; gaze at my baby in her crib; and finally walk downstairs to my waiting husband, knowing the long, romantic evening is ours—and it will be this way for many, many years.

Writing the Book

Sometimes I wonder what my life would be like if I'd had my children in my twenties. What if I'd decided that having a baby at forty was out of the question? For a moment, I try to imagine this foggy freedom. Surely I'd be taking martial arts classes and getting advanced degrees. I'd only go into the baby section at Target for shower gifts; and instead of knowing about every available item, I'd whisper to myself, "The things they come up with nowadays!" Nap times would be times I actually slept—not times I threw clothes in the washing machine or caught up on e-mail.

But then I come back to being a forty-year-old mother of a not-yet-crawling baby girl, and I know this is the life I want. You see, rather than anticipating a yoga class or an afternoon of leisurely shopping, I look forward to a first tooth, a first step, and a first word. Languidly stretched before me are wonderful, never-a-dull-moment days filled with Sunday-school dresses, school plays, and braces. What could be better?

At forty, so many chapters have been written in my book that I feel I've lived at least two lives. Now I get to open that book and tenderly teach my children from its pages, offering them instruction, guidance, patience, and joy. And I, who have lived so many lives already, get to rediscover the world: green trees and ocean breezes, the Constitution and the Holy Bible, Disney movies and mud pies.

Having a baby at forty is almost a paradox. I am quite old, and I have the wisdom to show for it. But that wisdom is only understood through eyes that see the world for the first time.

Afterthoughts on a Special Birth

The morning Leslie gave birth to Emma Grace, I sat huddled in the hospital waiting room with Leslie's mother-in-law, Lilly, and our friend Robin, our eyes glued to the television set. Parallel to Leslie's labor ran the panicked anguish of an entire nation. The date was September 11, 2001, and the unthinkable was unfolding before us. Lilly, Robin, and I had come to pray for, cheer on, and support Leslie in her hour of most intense need; but the shock of the terrorist attacks on New York City and Washington, D.C., kept jerking our focus and prayers in different directions. *What a time—what a day—to be having a midlife baby,* we thought.

Within minutes of Emma's delivery, we were allowed into the birthing room, just in time for the washing and weigh-in. Vowing not to spoil this precious once-in-her-lifetime moment, we didn't tell Leslie what was happening in the world outside. Nor did we tell her what was happening in the hospital halls, where doctors, nurses, aides, and visitors clumped around any TV they could find, glued to commentators frantic for words to describe the scenes on their studio monitors. In this little cocoon of a room, time stood still, and we purposefully basked in the glow of all that was still good and right in the world.

Later, in one of our church services, Leslie described her take on the fact that her long-anticipated midlife baby was born on one of the most infamous dates in American history.

"Emma's birth on such a tragic day for our country is, to me, a precious sign of healing, hope, and the goodness of God in the midst of despair," she said. "Every year on her birthday, she will be a picture to us of God's purposes, of how they prevail in spite of evil, and of the truth that his light will always pierce and overwhelm even the darkest night."

Never Say Never?

Many of the stroller-pushing midlife moms I've talked to are like Leslie. To them, their later-in-life baby is a wonderful gift from God. I don't doubt it. Yes, the new little ones keep them hopping—but in my book that translates into calories burned, muscles toned, energy boosted, and a really good chance that they'll still be thinking young when the rest of us are contemplating retirement. They may have gotten a late start; but from the looks of things, these late-blooming mothers will be in the race long past the rest of us.

Hmmm. Maybe I should…*naaah*. My hands are going to be plenty full just learning this grandmother thing.

Many, O LORD my God, are the wonders you have done. The things you planned for us no one can recount to you; were I to speak and tell of them, they would be too many to declare. (Ps. 40:5)

In the Chat Room

Janet, 51: *"I was forty when I found out I was pregnant with Bethany, our fourth child. While quite energetic and overachieving, she has also become my emotional mirror. When she hugs me or rubs my arm and says, 'Oh, Mom, I know how you feel,' I look into her ten-year-old eyes and know that she really does understand! I'm so grateful for my late-in-life baby."*

Kristy, 51: *"I was an 'oops' baby—born to my parents in their midlife. Now I'm my eighty-nine-year-old father's caregiver. Recently, as I was driving him to the doctor, Daddy said, 'Kristy, I remember when we found out your mother was expecting you, and we were so surprised. Times were hard for us, and it was a challenge. But I'm so thankful for you. You take such good care of me, and I love you so much.' I said, 'Daddy, remember all those times you took me to the pony rides and sat there and waited for*

140

me—and the horseback riding stables, and the public swimming pools, and the library, and all the other places? Well, as Mother used to say, "Turnabout's fair play." I love taking care of you.'"

Lindsey, 41: "I'm expecting our fifth baby any day—and this after a ten-year break. I thought I was done having babies, but then God began to tug at my heart. For two years I argued with him, 'But, God, you couldn't possibly mean to start all over again.' But he did. Following God is anything but boring! People assume by the space between my youngest and this pregnancy that this was an 'accident,' but no. I call her my 'radical obedience' baby."

Lisa, 45: "Our midlife baby has brought more joy to our family than we could have ever anticipated! She has given her grandmother new reasons to live. Our college-aged daughters want to attend schools that are close to home so they will be near Aimee as she grows up. And my husband and I feel and look younger and are highly motivated to stay in good shape."

Ellen, 42: "From the time I was old enough to talk, I said that I would never have children. My older brothers and I fought constantly, and that must have implanted the kids-are-nothing-but-trouble idea in my head. So after I got married, I waited for my heart to be softened...and waited. Finally, after sixteen years of marriage (and one vacation without birth control pills, which I neglected to pack), our beautiful, delightful daughter was born, and we can't imagine life without her."

Rhonda, 39: "I was carrying our infant daughter one evening when my husband asked how I would feel about him retiring at fifty. I told him, 'That would be great! You could help me carpool to grade school!' That freaked him out so much that he was completely unable to do the math. He said, 'Grade school? How old am I going to be when she gets out of college?' I told him, 'Sixty-one for undergrad school, and pushing up daisies if she goes to med school!'"

Mary, 38: "When a friend of mine became pregnant at thirty-five, she was a little anxious until I told her that my mom was thirty-five when I was born.

My friend said, 'Oh! And you turned out okay!' When I was growing up, younger mothers often sought my mom's advice. She stayed energetic and didn't start to age until I left home. I believe that having a younger offspring kept her younger than her peers. Having young children late in life can be a substitute for the fountain of youth."

Wynne, 79: "I had a baby when I was forty-two—actually my fourth natural child, but one who joined four wonderful stepchildren. The attending doctor mentioned that although I was his oldest patient, I was his easiest! Suffice it to say that we enjoyed that late baby, who was the eighth member of our family. She is now thirty-seven and expecting her fourth."

122 Things You Should Know by Now

You'd think that by this time in our lives, we surely would have learned *something*. And the truth is, we probably have accumulated more wisdom than we give ourselves credit for.

Want to know if you're on pace? Check yourself against this list of 122 things you should probably know by now:

1. *What to do with an artichoke*

2. *How to gargle, ladylike*

3. *How to make a small room look larger*

4. *How to make a large woman look smaller*

5. *What "abs," "pecs," and "glutes" are, and where they really belong*

6. *How to change the clock in your car*

7. *Who gets your chifforobe, commode, and four-poster bed if you don't happen to wake up in the morning*

8. *How to celebrate another woman's good news without thinking bad thoughts about her (or you)*

9. *How to wait for things*

10. *How to make real macaroni and cheese*

11. *How to clean and de-wrinkle anything made of silk*

12. *That a gentle answer turns away wrath*

13. *How to negotiate a win/win solution with anyone, anytime, anywhere, over anything*

14. *How to love the woman God made you to be*

15. *Your three greatest strengths*

16. *When it's okay to tell your mother no and not feel guilty*

17. *When to make your bed and when to let it go*

18. *Your all-time favorite movie*

19. *Your all-time favorite book*

20. *Your all-time favorite author*

21. *The next three books you plan to read*

22. *The five women you most admire and what intrigues you about them*

23. *The number of innings in a baseball game*

24. *How to live debt-free*

25. *How to have a rich time of solitude*

26. *How to take control of your mammogram*

27. *How to put gas in a car*

28. *How to take responsibility for your actions*

29. *How to live bitter-free*

30. *How to get a late checkout at a nice hotel*

31. *Your top three weaknesses and how to not be limited by them*

32. *What clothing styles best complement your body type*

33. *How to sing the national anthem aloud—and not care if anyone else does*

34. *How to stay calm if your credit card gets declined*

35. *How to get away for a couple of nights, alone, without fear that your husband, kids, or Foo-Foo the cat will starve to death*

36. *How to keep a checkbook in balance*

37. *How to introduce yourself to anyone, anytime, anywhere*

38. *What year your money market account will finally amount to something*

39. How to program a VCR

40. What colors you look good in besides black

41. The names of three people you would like to meet and at least one intelligent question you would ask each of them

42. How to send an e-mail with an attached document

43. The value of family reunions

44. How to do CPR

45. How to let your adult child make her own decisions without pitching a fit, resorting to pills, or pigging out in the pantry

46. What NFL stands for

47. How to relax with a half-finished to-do list

48. How and what to exfoliate

49. How to play at least one card game besides Go Fish

50. How to reduce night sweats and hot flashes by 80 percent

51. How to smile at people without giving them the wrong idea

52. How to say the Lord's Prayer and really mean it

53. How to work on self-defeating habits and attitudes with a pastor or professional counselor

54. Which cut flowers last the longest

55. How to wrap a gift in something more fun than mere wrapping paper

56. How to prepare a résumé

57. When you should compromise

58. When you should not compromise

59. How to write a letter to the editor

60. The hopes and dreams of the important people in your life

61. How to keep a meeting on task

62. How to ask for a raise and believe you are worth every penny of it

63. How to ask for forgiveness even though the other person was also at fault

64. Which interruptions are sent to you from heaven

65. How much life insurance your husband has and where he keeps important papers

66. How to host a smashing surprise party even if you've never been given one

67. How to make turkey gravy

68. How to keep a journal

69. The importance of resolving conflict now

70. How to make a cake for a baby shower out of disposable diapers

71. How to play charades

72. How to tell if a child is lying

73. How to make a genuine connection with God

74. How to give a bear hug

75. What to do with a first-aid kit

76. How to put out a fire without a fire extinguisher

77. How to pray for a miracle

78. How to be an encouragement to someone who has never thought to encourage you.

79. That less really is more

80. How to drive a stick shift

81. What a baby's cry means and what it takes to quiet it

82. How to make a moted sandcastle or a perfect sequence of snow angels

83. That a true friend cannot be won or lost

84. How to look natural on a horse

85. How to be a fun companion

86. How to use a FAX machine

87. How to say "thank you" after a compliment without feeling compelled to add, "But would you believe it only cost me $49.95?"

88. How to choose the most flattering, wearable swimsuit

89. That peace at all costs usually does

90. Where to dab concealer and where it won't do any good

91. How to know for sure that he's "the one"

92. How to be content even though everything that used to be no longer is

93. How to make a romantic meatloaf

94. That with God, all things are possible

95. The best time of year to buy living-room furniture

96. How to ask for help from anyone, anytime, anywhere, for anything

97. Where to get a great massage

98. That everyone deserves a second chance (unless someone's life is in danger)

99. How to get the best seat on a commercial airplane

100. That your parents didn't do everything wrong

101. How to find information on the Internet

102. *How to face the facts*

103. *That the position does not make the person—the person makes the position*

104. *How to pack for a week in one carry-on bag*

105. *How to do a breast self-exam*

106. *How to take one thing at a time*

107. *What you want to be now that you are all grown up*

108. *How to choose the right lip liner*

109. *That makeup is not essential for a good workout and will only clog your pores*

110. *How to eat alone in a restaurant and be fully entertained*

111. *How to leave room each day for spontaneity*

112. *That people are rarely as good as they say they are or as bad as we think they are*

113. *That people are more important than things*

114. *That people are more important than projects*

115. *That people are more important than programs*

116. *That people are more important than profits*

117. *That no matter what we do, we're all in the people business*

118. *That joy does not need a reason*

119. *That wisdom is greater than knowledge*

120. *That love demands a high cost, but chilled is the heart without it*

121. *The sound of God's voice in the dark*

122. *Three precious gifts you bring to the world*

PART 4

I Will Survive and Thrive

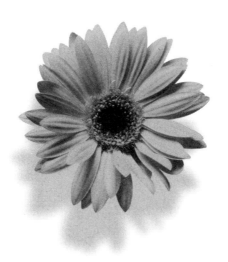

16

Instead of drowning in change
or just treading water to keep our
heads above its surface,
we can make art of the churn.
—Candice Carpenter

Restocking the Empty Nest

Many factors determine how intense our empty-nest syndrome will be. For some moms, watching the kids drive off is an exhilarating, anticipated time. For some, it brings a sigh of relief. Then there are the moms on the other extreme—the ones for whom the phrase *grief-stricken* only begin to describe the exit wounds. Whatever our take on this experience—just one more of midlife's transitions—the wisest among us say to ourselves, *This is your time…see the possibilities…seek new ways to fill the gaps…put to fresh use your previously spoken-for finances…spend your energy on people and things that will last.*

New Purchasing Power

One of the real advantages of an empty nest is that money previously spent to feed voracious teenage appetites and buy new Nikes every four months is now available for all those things you put off buying for twenty-some years. For example:

A new car. My good friend Pam recently bought a snazzy European sports car. Her youngest had just gone off to college, and since the lease was up on her old car, she and her husband looked at each other and said, "Why not?" They call it their "empty-nester car," which is an accurate description since you can only get two people in it. Of course, restocking your nest with a purchase like this requires a sizable investment and a serious preference for the windblown look. So far, the best I've been able to do is to downsize my American-made minivan to a midsize Japanese model. But, hey, it's a start.

Jewelry. Recently I read a magazine article in which a woman stated that her jewelry purchases have ramped up quite a bit since she entered midlife. This made sense to me, since many people are at the peak of their earning potential at this point and can better afford the expense. But the woman said the reason *she* buys more jewelry is not because she can afford it, but because it makes her feel prettier. According to her, jewelry draws attention to itself and away from her wrinkles and crow's feet.

A second home. Some couples are able to buy additional property after the kids leave, but there seems to be a split decision as to the motive. A man is likely to choose to buy a ski condo or beach house merely for the investment. But a woman will encourage the purchase because she knows it will make excellent bait to lure the kids home for a visit.

Cosmetics. Recent years have witnessed a sharp increase in the purchase of cosmetics for the middle-aged: wrinkle creams, antioxidant lotions, under-eye concealers, and special vitamin-packed "cosmeceuticals" targeted to fight the effects of aging. One forty-something woman I know recently confessed she has just *now*, for the first time *ever*, started wearing foundation. So for her, all the money she will soon find herself spending on makeup will be a real shock-in-the-purse.

Of course, we all know about the scores of women who are opting for various degrees of cosmetic surgery. My good friend Martha has this message for any readers currently considering "alterations." "Tell everyone *not* to get plastic surgery. That way, those of us who don't want to, won't look so bad in comparison!"

New Hobbies and Interests

Remember all those hobbies and interests you said you'd pick up, if only you had the time? Well, now that your nest is empty, you no longer have an excuse. Why not give one of these a try:

Skydiving. One woman I know celebrated her fiftieth birthday by leaping out of an airplane at fifteen thousand feet. (It's truly sad, the effect middle age has on some women.) After watching the video of her jump, I can think of about ten zillion better ways to celebrate my birthday outside the box. But if skydiving, parasailing, or the latest parachute-wearing sport, *parasail surfing*, is something that really piques your interest—I recommend that you get your heart and your head examined first. Then go for it.

Cooking classes. My family would roll on the floor in a fit if they knew, but I have actually thought about attending a cooking class. Emeril makes it look fun. Martha makes it look easy.

Sometimes I imagine that I could be the calm, lovely hostess of one of those New England-style, come-as-you-are cookouts, where the table decor is plucked fresh from a nearby woods and forty of your closest friends stand around the backyard tossing low-fat salads. The problem is, I don't live in New England, and I'm pretty sure the entire mosquito population of the Southeast is headquartered in my neighborhood. And besides, I wouldn't know a leek if it dripped on me.

So, on second thought, maybe cooking wouldn't pan out for me. But you might fare much better. Why not start a monthly Diners Club, or try a few Dinner-and-DVD get-togethers with like-nested friends?

Reading. Books stimulate the mind (which you already know from reading this one) and they entertain (which this author thinks is okay as long as you are careful to occasionally expose yourself to more serious works of literature). The truth is, reading is like sit-ups for the brain; according to the experts, it's exactly the kind of exercise people need as they mature. (For once, this author and the experts are one.)

Why not start a monthly book club? If you do, let me recommend two not-to-be-missed classics for female readers: *The Grass Is Always Greener over the Septic Tank* by Erma Bombeck and *Leaking Laffs between Pampers and Depends* by Barbara Johnson. You can even make your club mobile by taking a trip to the town or setting of the book your group is reading. If you decide to bring your group to Orlando (which is, of course, the illustrious setting of this book), I will be happy to arrange a brief tour of the kitchen where, on a daily basis, Hero the dog barks at the refrigerator until someone gets him an ice cube.

Tracing your genealogy. If you like history, research, and have a computer, tracing your family tree is a great hobby. Our friends

Ginny and Bernard are serious "tracers" who went so far as to draw their tree on a wall in their home. They've also made trips to the towns where Bernard's ancestors lived. I have a theory that many of us get more interested in learning about our fore-parents the closer we get to actually meeting them.

Traveling. More and more people go cruising in midlife—no, not the thing you used to do in high school. I mean actually voyaging to exotic ports of call.

For our twenty-fifth anniversary, David and I took our first cruise to Alaska. One night was designated "formal night," and everyone strolled the promenade deck in swank tuxedos and beaded gowns while trying hard not to think about certain unfortunate scenes from the movie *Titanic.* My biggest fear, though, wasn't icebergs; it was gaining more weight. Cruise ships are famous for their all-you-can-eat, twenty-four-hours-a-day buffets. Then our steward mentioned a little known dietary fact shared only among those in the cruising industry: Ninety-five percent of all people breathing salt air on an ocean liner will actually burn more calories than those breathing regular city air. After the trip David and I concluded that (a) we were among the 5 percent who failed to benefit from this phenomenon, and (b) on our next cruise, we won't believe everything we hear.

Writing. As you know by now, this is my category. I began writing professionally when my boys were in high school. A little at a time, when I wasn't involved in various ministries, I took classes, attended writers' conferences, and began submitting short manuscripts to innocent, unsuspecting magazines. To my amazement it wasn't long before my first book, *Hugs from Heaven: Embraced by the Savior,* was published.

Lots and lots of writers begin their careers at the halfway

point. Julia Child wrote her first cookbook at the age of forty-nine. It's not too late for you to start now.

If writing for the public sounds too intimidating, however, consider writing your personal memoirs. Think about it: How often have you wished that you knew more about your grandmother or great-grandmother's life? Wouldn't it have been great if they had written down some of the fascinating details of their lives? Your daily adventures might not seem noteworthy to you right now, but in fifty years much of what we know of modern life will have gone the way of all other dinosaurs. Your little ol' memoirs could become a significant resource for your great-great-granddaughter as she sits in a boat in Lake Michigan while taking an online tour of the Smithsonian Institute with the rest of her virtual class.

If you're going to write a personal history, though, now is the time to begin—while you've still got some memory and can question siblings and friends on the accuracy of events. Book-stores have tons of resources on how to get started. Writing your memories is not only a great pastime, it's a great way to trace the grace of God in your life and give testimony to the next generations of the power of Christ to change and sustain those who follow him.

Making a Change

One of the few constants in life—and particularly midlife—is *change*. If you've ever thought of making some big changes, now is the time to do it.

Changing your career. A lot of women change jobs, start small businesses, or find creative ways to alter their job descriptions at midlife. Some, when they wake up to the fact that they're not getting any younger, decide that enjoying life is more important than working overtime. To them, job satisfaction, or finding and doing something they're passionate about, is worth certain monetary sacrifices. Other women feel they have only so much earning time left, so they ramp up their workloads and time sheets. Both approaches are understandable. My conclusion is this: Some of us will work less, while others will work more. Do whatever *works* for you.

Going back to school. This is a favorite option for many women who primarily worked at home while their kids were growing up. They suddenly realize there are many things about life they simply must find out about! Some are eager to get the background they need to go back into the work force—you know, the same work force that droves of tired, middle-aged men are in the process of getting out of. (Hopefully we can make this stampede of a personnel switch in an orderly fashion, without anyone getting hurt.) Some women, in their postmenopausal zest, find enough energy to work during the day and go to school at night. Personally, I'm asking God to pass me by with so much zest.

Meeting the parents—again. Many of us may soon discover what it's like to live with our parents again after thirty or forty years of living in separate locations. As their health declines, our parents are likely to need us more than ever, and the best option for many of us will be to move Mom or Dad into that bedroom that was recently vacated. Minus the posters, of course.

Remember the old TV show *The Waltons?* The grandparents always lived in the same house with their children and grandchildren, so when it came time for middle-age care giving, no big adjustment was necessary. Maybe they were on to something; because for most of us, a live-in care situation means a radical, sweeping change. Just deciding who's in charge—who the "real" parent is—can be a tough issue to tackle. Once we work the kinks out, however, the result (as many now report) can be a wonderful time of rebonding as we prayerfully and gracefully give back to the ones who gave so much to us.

Getting Involved

While we're on the subject of giving back, midlife (as you have no doubt heard from a number of sources by now) really is a great time to invest in others—and glorify God in the process.

Community volunteering. With the kids out of the house, you now have more time to build houses with Habitat for Humanity, take short-term mission trips with Youth with a Mission, or help your local Meals on Wheels deliver warm lunches to the elderly. What about volunteering at your grandchild's school (or any school in your neighborhood) as a reader or mentor? The Red Cross always needs people to help with emergencies somewhere in the world; if you can't leave town, you can at least donate a few pints of blood. Hospitals need volunteers to do magic tricks for kids, give directions, push people around in wheelchairs, steer library and flower carts, and generally help sick people smile more so they get can get well faster.

Church volunteering. A really good place to offer your services is your local church. Chances are very high they need telephones answered, babies rocked, children mentored, students challenged, women encouraged, Bible studies taught, catering arranged, landscaping dug, weddings planned, cleaning supplied, offerings given, guests greeted or housed, and choirs filled. And the great extra value of volunteering at church is that every bit of the time, talent, and treasure you give transfers beautifully into the Next Life.

Starting a new ministry. What issues or areas are you most passionate about? The arts? Latchkey children? Troubled teens? Abused women? Cooking? Literacy? Homemaking? Parenting? Leadership? Bible Study? Prayer? Missions? Mentoring and discipleship? Talk to church leaders and see what needs are out there that you may be gifted to meet. If you tend to be better at behind-the-scenes, organizational tasks, team up with a teacher-type or some other up-front person who has the same passion you do. Ask yourself how many hours a week you would be willing to invest in the lives of others for the sake of Christ. What would you be willing to do, even in a small way?

Think about how Christ has transformed your life, then think about what ministry may be missing from your local church or community. What area do you keep thinking about, always saying to yourself, *Someone really needs to do something about that?* Perhaps that's the prompting of the Holy Spirit, trying to birth a new way of caring for the people God loves *through you.*

Giving Our Hearts Away

There's no question that for many women, the transitional days of empty nesting will have moments that are neither happy nor exhilarating. They will be more like times of mourning. As women, as sisters, we need to be sensitive to each other, observant and aware of the challenges our friends and coworkers face in this area, offering to listen, comfort, and, when necessary, pass the tissues.

But ultimately, as the echoes from our empty homes trail off, we need to encourage one another to take the quickest, most proven way back to purpose and joy in life: finding new, fulfilling ways to open our hearts—and then, one little piece at a time, giving them away.

Sow your seed in the morning, and at evening let not your hands be idle. (Eccles. 11:6)

In the Chat Room

Anne, 48: *"My husband and I have a little money now. We can leave the kids at home when we take trips and have more time to concentrate on each other."*

Shirlee, 51: *"When the kids left home, my husband and I realized how much our arguing had centered around them. I would like to travel more internationally; I've been to twenty-three countries and have one hundred or so more to go. I would love to work in a gift shop and be a grandma."*

Jackie, 46: *"I enjoy my job. I would like to expand my education and get my degree, then move into more of an educator role in my field."*

Joann, 59: *"Someday I would love to work full time in a children's ministry. But I remind myself daily to serve the Lord where I am. I would also love to sail and travel more."*

Martha, 49: *"I love not having a career and being involved in my husband's ministry. I have enough interests to enable me to fill my time with things I enjoy and feel purpose about. I plan on pursuing painting."*

Susan, 49: *"I love my career as a kindergarten teacher. I get great fulfillment from loving and teaching and encouraging children. But I'd love to travel more and run a marathon."*

Shirley, 40: *"I want to know where we're headed in the next twenty years. My husband says I'm having a midlife crisis, but I think it's important to plan ahead. We need to look at doing some things together so we don't draw apart. I'm feeling like I'm running out of time to do the things I have left to do. I want to learn the bagpipes and travel to Alaska and Canada."*

Mary Lou, 51: *"I wasn't prepared for midlife. I didn't read or prepare mentally for personal and family changes. But I like my age now. I feel I've experienced a number of things—like travel, education, and faith—that keep me looking forward and moving ahead."*

Books to Help You Remodel Your Nest

Chapters: Create a Life of Exhilaration and Accomplishment in the Face of Change by Candice Carpenter

What's Next? Women Redefining Their Dreams in the Prime of Life by Rena Pederson with Dr. Lee Smith

The Mentor Quest: Practical Ways to Find the Guidance You Need by Betty Southard

Growing Young: Embracing the Joy and Accepting the Challenges of Mid-Life by Lois Mowday Rabey

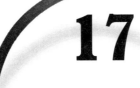

17

Animals are such agreeable friends,
they ask no questions,
they pass no criticisms.
—George Eliot

Midlife Goes to the Dogs

Okay, so the kids are growing up and moving on. In the last chapter, we discussed a number of safe, fun, soul-flooding ways to replenish the cavernous void created when the children leave home. But there is one other option. And statistics show it will likely involve an animal.

That's right. A survey by the Ralston-Purina Company a couple of years ago revealed that 57 percent of pet owners were forty years old or above. And 60 percent of the pet owners surveyed said there were no children under eighteen in the house.[1] Which means, if you don't own a pet at the moment you can expect a strange, magnetic hankering for one sometime within the next six months.

It also means pets are taking over the world.

If you have ever surfed the vast array of animal-lover channels on TV, you know it's true. Every minute of every day from now till the cows come home, you can find at least one program in which a guy in a safari suit is darting through the jungle singing the praises of deadly snakes and man-eating crocodiles. Who needs *Monday Night Football* when you can opt for the "Canine Olympics," with brown and white collies running obstacle courses, and zealous color commentators replaying their every leap and stride?

Sweet as they may be, and as necessary as some claim they are to a balanced global ecology, I am not a big animal fan, domesticated or otherwise. And when my kids all fly the coop, I for one have no plans to pour out my last remaining cup of human kindness on some yippity-yapping, four-legged mongrel. I have legitimate reasons for taking this stand: smells, slobber, and pooper-scoopers, for starters. But the biggest reason by far is a dog named Yogi.

(Violins please.)

Pardon My Dog

When I was in second grade, my stepmother (whom we believed to be of sound mind) drove down to the Humane Society and, without fair warning, pardoned a dog that, in my opinion, should have remained on death row. For reasons known only to her, Mom's choice was a mid-sized, black and white terrier—a breed whose name, if you really think about it, sounds suspiciously like the word *terror*. Someone named this dog Yogi, after the cartoon bear, which was way too nice a moniker for the snap-happy, kid-hating, attack mutt he turned out to be.

After only a few days, it was clear that Yogi was not smarter than your average dog. He refused to sit or fetch. He was not the least bit interested in wearing doll clothes, and he maimed any-one (except Mom) who tried to pick him up. To his credit, Yogi did a good job of keeping himself and our floor licked clean, and he was faithful to tell us when the mail had arrived. But when Yogi was around, you pretty much had to watch your back and keep on his good side—like you would if you went swimming in a shark tank or happened upon a grizzly in the wild. And after about fourteen years, this arrangement got kind of old.

Thanks to Yogi, I have never, ever been a dog person.

Unfortunately, my son Jonathan grew up with a dog obses-sion. "When I get older, I'm gonna get a truck and a dog," he'd announce. Or he'd say, "Mom, don't you think if ever a boy needed a dog, it's me?"

But no matter what angle he tried, I was firm: "Honey, I'm sorry. I hate to disappoint you. But we are just not a pet-type family." I was not about to add the upkeep of a hungry, howling hound to all my other responsibilities. Absolutely no pets. Ever.

Who Let the Dog In?

Fast-forward ten years.

Warning: It is never—I repeat, never—a smart idea to leave a nineteen-year-old, especially a dog-deprived nineteen-year-old, unattended while you and your husband go off on a roman-tic ten-day vacation. Kids at this age think they can do just about anything. They have their own money. They are, for the most part, legal; and because they know that you know they will soon be striking out on their own, they are likely to take advantage of your weakened, vulnerable state.

And so it was that David and I returned, rested and refreshed, from a blissful time away together, just the two of us (a luxurious freedom that has to be one of, if not the most, glorious benefits of marriage at midlife). Anxious for a joyous reunion with our sons, we burst through the door—only to be mauled by an out-of-control, yippity-yapping, saliva-dripping puppy.

I went numb. Surely it isn't...surely he didn't...but one look from Jon, and I knew. While we were off lounging by the Pacific, all starry-eyed and clueless, the boy who used to be our son was combing the Humane Society in search of the happiest, healthiest, hugest dog he could find.

And the lot fell to Hero.

By the time we got home, the damage had been done. There was a dog dish in the laundry room, a crate beside Jon's bed, and chew toys under the table. Hero had already been clipped, dipped, and snipped. And our son had a new best friend.

"We can take him back if you don't like him, Mom."

"He gets exactly one week to prove himself, Jon, and so help me, if one single thing in this house gets torn up...."

It has now been nine months.

When Jon is out late, which, naturally, is almost every night, Hero sleeps on the floor at the foot of our bed (or when it suits him, on top of it). He has ripped a hole in the porch screen big enough to climb through, chewed the corners off my best rug, and deposited a certain odor in every room that I swore I'd never have in my house.

Without a photo it's hard to appreciate him, but try to

imagine a butterscotch-brown, Labrador-Rotweiller-German Shepherd combo-dog with an intriguing face that cocks in a funny way when he's trying to figure out what you want him to do.

He has not officially been to "school," so he jumps on people, and when no one is looking, he stands on his hind legs and swipes biscuits off the counter. He's supposed to sit in his crate when he's been bad, but that seems cruel; so I banish him to the backyard, where he flits around chasing dragonflies and chewing up the bushes.

Our house is mostly quiet during the day now. The calls and shouts of little boys are gone; no basketballs bounce on the driveway, no one wrestles in the hall or slides mattresses down the stairs. I really miss those sounds.

But it is not entirely quiet here. Again, thanks to Jonathan. We still have a generous supply of gnawing, whacking, clicking, barking, crunching, slurping, snorting, and tag jingling to keep us company.

Who Lets the Dog in Now?

I get up from the computer again. Milk chocolate eyes peer at me through the paw-printed glass door, while a giant tail whacks the air. Someone wants in where the people are. As the door slides open, I ask Hero if he wants a drink of water. He says not really, he's good for now. Then he sprawls on the floor, next to my desk, keeping watch as I write.

When David comes home, Hero will bolt for the door, and I will tell David about the dog's exploits in almost the same way I used to report the daily antics of our sons. Then David will get out the leash and take our charge for a walk, and while they're gone, I will get out the mop and wash the dirt marks off the kitchen floor for the third time this week.

It must be midlife madness. How else do you explain it?

The whole world has gone to the dogs.

👀 In the Chat Room

Trish, 52: *"A few years ago, when I was going through a divorce, I bought a little dog, thinking that she would be a happy distraction for my daughters. But before long the girls were off to college, I remarried, and Tootsie became mine. I can't tell you what an unbelievably calming effect she has on me, especially those nights (which are many) when I can't sleep, and my mind is racing and fidgety. That's when I go downstairs with a book, and Tootsie climbs on the couch and curls up next to me. I can't really explain it, but she's a wonderful constant at this time in my life."*

Lauren, 44: *"Although the decision to purchase Sophie, our teacup poodle, was made on a whim, I had been aware for quite some time that our family dynamics could change any minute. Our three daughters were growing up faster than I had imagined; and, sure enough, within a few months of getting the dog, our oldest daughter was engaged. The exodus is beginning now. But Sophie will stay here with me."*

Kathy, 48: *"The newness of being in that group of 'people who have pets' still hasn't worn off, even though it's been almost a year since Muggsie arrived. While we wait for grandchildren, our funny-faced, four-legged bundle of joy is bringing us countless hours of entertainment and laughter."*

Hope in God, who richly provides us with everything for our enjoyment. (1 Tim. 6:17)

18

Normal day, let me be aware of the
treasure you are. Let me learn
from you, love you,
bless you before you depart.
—Mary Jean Iron

A Month in the
Middle of Life

Day 1

Made a big decision today. Because my body is God's temple; because I need strength, energy, and stamina to do the work he has called me to; because I want to "be there" for my husband, children, and soon-coming grandchild and don't want to exit before my time is up; because I have reached the size of a refrigerator, and creative camouflage has lost all effectiveness—for all these reasons, I will start today to transform my lifestyle and go on a no-sugar, high-protein, low-carb, high-water diet with medium intense cardio exercise five days a week and moderate weight training three. Will start eating legal fruit and raw carrots whenever I get the slightest urge for such things as White Chocolate Chunk Hawaiian Macadamia Nut Surprise Cookies, which are on the second shelf in the pantry (left over from last Tuesday's midlife support group). Weight loss goal: thirty pounds in a month (will settle for eight).

Day 2

Pulled together and filled out all of Joseph's graduation paraphernalia. (Who designs these forms?) Paid extra for the bells and whistles. Why not? This is our last and final high school graduation, which is something I am determined to keep rational about. It's only a life-altering, every-day-changing, entire-family-impacting event that I *could* make a scene over. Have made up my mind to attend with my heart on a tight leash.

Day 3

Observed for the first time a strange, new puffiness in the midriff area. Very upsetting. Was already distraught about back fat, thigh fat, rear fat, ab fat, and face fat. Never, ever had this kind of fat. Determined not to let it get me down. Did two full sets of ten modified ab crunches as shown in a magazine in the grocery store checkout line.

Day 4

Actually had an inkling of a thought concerning the potential of a romantic encounter with my beloved sometime in the near future.

Day 5

Made an appointment with the eye doctor. Am also weighing the pros and cons of getting a chiropractic adjustment for the throbbing back pain caused by holding all reading material at arm's length for the last year and a half.

Day 6

On top of my usual Phyto-Estrogen and Super-Mega-Extra-Potency-Multivitamin for Women, began taking vitamin C-Ester, vitamin E, Alpha Lipoic Acid, DMAE, Coenzyme Q-10, and Tums PMS to improve skin tone, tighten elasticity, and fight those raging free radicals.

Day 7

Noticed even more feet deformity due to bunions. Have serious, pronounced slanting of toes and toenails, but can still walk without assistance. Not bad enough to warrant surgery. Effective immediately, will try wearing pedicure toe separators to bed and just see what happens.

Day 8

Finally went for a mammogram. Wasn't as bad as I'd thought. Yeah! Discovered one situation in which a small cup size is actually preferable.

Day 9

Very unhappy with my hair. Thin. Color-fried ends. Style less than fresh. Can't seem to find an easy-to-manage haircut that will work with my fleshy, oval face and pear-shaped body. Time to break out the Yellow Pages and change hairstylists again.

Day 10

Enjoyed a nice lunch with my sisters until we got on the subject of my upcoming birthday. Great fun was had by all at my expense. Sadly, both sisters must now forfeit their invites to the festivities and will be cast in a less than lovely light in my soon-to-be-published novel, *When We Were Family*.

Day 11

Had been basking in the sweet revelation that, with Joseph getting a car for graduation, I finally have a vehicle to myself after all these years of sharing cars with teenagers. Then Jon announced today he has to sell his car in order to square some mounting debts. I'm proud of his decision and sorry for his sacrifice. Offered the use of my car for a while. God's timing makes me smile. Can't leave the house anyway for at least a month—not until I finish this book.

Day 12

Decided to eat only salmon, lettuce, and strawberries. Will wait to see if there's really a noticeable improvement in my skin tone, weight, and memory.

Day 13

It's déjà vu all over again. Started birth control pills today. Haven't taken them in twenty-six years. Doctor says it's perfectly safe, since there are no major female cancer issues in my family. Says they should help bring everything back in order for me, or just about. The guys in the house will be happy. If all goes well, Mom can stop hogging the Clearasil.

Day 14

Got eyebrows waxed and was a hair away from saying go ahead, do the chin too, but chickened out. Once you start, there's no turning back.

Also, for the record, there is no disgrace in starting a meal plan over again. It's when you stop starting over that you should really start worrying.

Day 15

Led singing for a meeting at church and sounded pathetic. Breathing is off—way shallow. Actually felt ashamed of my voice for the first time in my adult life. It's my fault for not keeping it in shape. Plenty of women much older than me still have excellent singing voices. So what's my problem?

Day 16

Feeling very guilty today. Eight months have passed, and we still don't have a marker on Mom's grave. We're still paying for the funeral—and had no idea grave markers were so expensive. All this time Mom has laid out there in the Tomb for the Unknown Woman. If we don't hurry up, the grass is going to grow in, and we won't be able to tell which side of Daddy she's buried on. One thing's for sure: She wouldn't have let any of us lay out there unaccounted for like that. If money were an issue, she would have at least had a garage sale. For now Daddy will just have to share his nameplate with Mom—which, if you think about it, sounds like something a husband wouldn't mind doing for his wife, even if it has been thirty-three years since they've seen each other.

Day 17

Jon's dog, Hero, chewed a chunk out of my Bible this morning. It was lying out on the kitchen counter, and, apparently, since no one was paying attention to him, Hero decided to take the perceived slight out on God. Genesis and Exodus are completely gone now. I suppose if you have to lose part of your Bible, those are two books you could manage to go without for a little while.

Am still waiting to see if Hero gets a sudden urge to wander. If he does, I, for one, will not stop him, since this is not his first offense.

Day 18

Became aware today of a frightening new habit: I'm actually walking around the house in the middle of the day, fully clothed, wearing my bedroom shoes. Never liked how this looked when Mom did it, but have to admit I can hardly think of a more comfortable feeling of late. Still...

Day 19

Last night we stayed home, put our feet up, and watched the classic movie channel—again. Wondering this morning if this sudden shift from going out to staying in should concern us more, but neither of us seems to feel we are missing much. It's nice to be carefree—no dressing up, fighting traffic, waiting in line for a table, racing for a good seat at the movies. Probably should do more with other people, but even that requires more gas than we've got some nights.

Day 20

Am sure I have missed my period this month. First time in thirty-seven years this has happened (except when I was pregnant or nursing). Probably have about a 1 percent chance of pregnancy, but seriously doubt it in light of other key factors. Fully expected that brooding and sadness would overtake me at this milestone, but so far they have not come. Wonder if they will.

Day 21

Bought another new exercise outfit, hoping to juice up some motivation.

Day 22

Still not comfortable wearing glasses at church. Totally prideful of me. What's the big deal? I don't even blink when other people wear their glasses.

Day 23

To help Becca with ideas, bought several books about decorating a baby's room. Had fun dreaming. Then prayed for God to help me remember that this is *her* pregnancy, *her* baby, and *her* baby's room.

Only two-and-a-half months to go—and still have no earthly idea how to be a grandmother. Prayed for God to help me have a more positive outlook on the prospect.

Day 24

Am convinced I sensed a genuine tinge of amorous inclination toward David but was way too tired and decided it best not to broadcast it.

Day 25

Fell off the salmon wagon. Gave in to burger and fries. They were too convenient. Not a complete glutton, though, since I scraped off the mayonnaise and cheese. Later remembered a stash of Tootsie Rolls in the pantry. Did four of those. I don't even like Tootsie Rolls.

Day 26

Today Joshua, Becca, and baby Gavin-still-under-construction flew to that church near Chicago where they've been offered a staff position. I know it's a good church, and I know we're all in the body of Christ, but I'm still in denial here. Best thing is to make my heart go neutral. But it won't go, and at the moment I don't have the strength to force it. I want what I want. And what I want is for them to stay here, to let us mentor them in parenting, to let us learn how to bounce a grandchild on our knees on a regular basis, and so much more. It would save a whole lot of tears if God would be in favor of my idea of a perfect, happy family—and if he'd convince them too.

Day 27

Finally discovered the mystery mildew smell: Joseph's athletic shoes. Started to send him out with the credit card, then remembered that my days of shoe buying for teenagers have nearly expired. Gave Joe a choice to head to the mall on his own, or take Mom along. He chose me! Consciously worked at savoring that moment, and had lots of great conversation on the way. Joe raked in two pairs of shoes, jeans, a pair of shorts, and socks. Mom bagged one more memory.

Day 28

New, deep-cut wrinkle has appeared on the left side of my chin under my mouth. Looks like a scar from a knife fight. How do these show up overnight? Turned an aging corner with this one, I think. Wish I'd known sooner that sugar fast-forwards a woman's face. Guess I better start sleeping faceup.

Day 29

Lost another two pounds for the third time this month.

Day 30

While waiting for my teeth to whiten (thought I'd try one of those new, over-the-counter whitening systems), got out the family album and looked at old photos. Did a few instant replays in my mind. Was touched again in that place where the sight of a little boy's stubby body pricks a momma's heart. There has never been such a family. Anywhere. Ever.

Day 31

Thinking back over the last thirty days and feeling thankful. All in all, I would give this month a B. B for the Bending it required at times. And for the Bewilderment. Even for things Bittersweet. For the Blendings, the Blessings, and the moments of marital Bliss. For the Blues. And even for the Bon voyages.

I give it a B for my three sometimes Brash, sometimes Bashful Boys. For Bodies in Bonus with Babies. For Bridges reaching. For Brightness and Breath. For the Benefits of Being a Believer. But mostly I give it a B because…I'm Becoming.

In the Chat Room

Martha, 49: "*Some days I have more confidence, and some days I feel like an old lady. It's hard not to focus on the newly forming wrinkles, sags, and fat pockets.*"

Anne, 48: "*I like parenting at this stage. The kids are more fun. I enjoy and appreciate the fact that I won't have them around much longer. I've tried to pull away and not get as involved in their lives. I'm trying to encourage them to make more decisions on their own.*"

Susan, 49: *"My faith makes me see the good in every season."*

Lisa, 47: *"Midlife is something I'm somewhat confused about. I'm not quite sure how I'm supposed to be feeling or how it affects me. I guess it's a-learn-as-you-go type of thing. No one warned me of the internal changes I would be going through. It's like I'm trying to figure out what's going on and what I need to do about it. Doctors don't know, and books are contradictory."*

Suzie, 52: *"I think it helps to find a friend who is going through the same thing. You can laugh about stuff and empathize about the hard parts. Our hormones affect everything. It's very important to be able to express feelings without being judged."*

Shirlee, 51: *"I'm very much 'in-process,' still trying to figure out what I think and feel and what all this means to me spiritually and career-wise."*

Lauren, 44: *"I am more high maintenance now. I have to spend more time and money on myself. It doesn't really bother me, though, because my friends are going through it too. There's safety in numbers."*

Laurie, 37: *"I try to surround myself with other women who are going through the same things. We laugh and cry together. I try to take care of myself, pamper myself once in a while. For me, a good haircut really helps."*

My days are swifter than a weaver's shuttle.... Remember, O God, that my life is but a breath. (Job 7:6–7)

Tracking a Month in the Middle of Your Life

On index cards or in a small spiral notebook, prenumber Days 1 through 31. Each day write down one or two "snapshots" that capture an experience or subject that presents itself to you. Keep it short, or you won't follow through. This is different than journaling. Think telegram size.

The benefits? I discovered at least four:

- You begin to pay better attention to your life.

- You learn to identify and savor special moments.

- You track habits, trends, and thoughts that you can dissect and contemplate later.

- You capture and store a slice of your everyday life, so you can go back and remind yourself of the unique season you've been through.

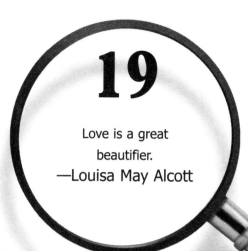

19

Love is a great
beautifier.
—Louisa May Alcott

I Think I Can Face the Music, If Someone Will Dance with Me

When we were first married, whenever I would visualize David and me together in our later years, it was always in a sort of American Gothic picture: two very old people rocking on a front porch or walking hand in hand in a park, flanked by greedy pigeons. For whatever reason, I never saw us midstream—never imagined what we might look like or how we might act when we got to where we are now.

There is a smooth roundedness to our relationship (not to mention our bodies) now, like two grayish stones at the edge of a wild river gorge. A lot of water has washed over these rocks and, over time, worn down a fair amount of sharpness and pride. We seem to have found our groove. By far, it's the best place we've been as a couple. But the fact that we've "arrived" is a reality we're both still adjusting to.

When All You Can Do Is Laugh

At times I've been anxious about my waning features—that frightful moving of the old, familiar me into the new, next me. Then I look at David and see a similar remodeling going on, and it makes me smile. We share the annoyance of fuzzy eyesight and the irritation of forgetting our glasses (since they are such new appliances). Now when I get in David's face, it turns blurry; and I wonder if God, in his compassionate intentionality, has not secretly arranged for our vision to go at the same pace as our youthfulness.

We joke (a little nervously) about the changes. We have weird growths on our faces—wartish looking moles that seem to pop up overnight. Sometimes we stand in front of the bathroom mirror doing bump competitions to see who has the most new ones. There is more face flesh than before, and that bothers us to no end. We keep wondering: *Are we ever going to lose enough weight to make that extra jaw line disappear?*

I poke fun at his missing hair, and he scolds me for all the falling-out gray ones that keep clogging the shower drain. And a funny thing happens when we hug now. Different parts of us touch first—a new thing just this year—and while it disturbs us on the one hand, it's laughable, too, like a pair of belly-bumping athletes after an extra fine play.

David's back has "gone out" several times in the last few years—an event previously unthinkable for such a healthy man who's never known a limitation on his body. As a result, we aren't as free to do just anything anymore; we have to consider if it will set him back. And most nights when the boys come home late, they are treated to the sight of their mom sprawled on the family room couch, getting her aching feet rubbed. I think of all the old people I've met who have little else to talk about but their latest pain or ailment, and I wonder, *Is this the beginning of that for us?*

Great Honking Jackhammers

Earlier we talked about the challenge of sleeping with a wet-mop insomniac. But in the last year, David and I have been forced to deal with another of the really great nocturnal aggravations: snoring.

When the big honks first began, we had about a sixty-forty chance of hitting a non-snore night. Now it's more like twenty-eighty. Not only do I have to fight night sweats, sleeplessness, and bathroom breaks, I'm also forced to battle Slumberjack Dave. This bothers me so much that I recently turned to the Internet for help. What I discovered was an alarming epidemic of nasal deformities creating an avalanche of marital chaos—all over the world.

I saw one message board that read, "My husband, largely due to being overweight, has a terribly loud snoring problem, which has caused us to sleep apart just so I can rest. His attitude of 'live with it' is aggravating and makes me resentful, and his refusal to attempt any remedy has caused a strain on our twenty-eight-year marriage. We are currently in therapy to address this."

A man then posted this reply: "Noise suppression earplugs, that's what you need. They're used to protect hearing in noisy industrial situations. I buy them by the box. I think they cost about fifty cents a pair and can be washed and reused a couple of times."

So earplugs are a possible solution. According to one Web site, I can also sew a tennis ball on the back of David's pajama shirt (if he wore one) like they did for the soldiers in World War I. Or I can buy him an electric shock wristband that wakes him up every time he snores. The only problem is I'm afraid of getting shocked myself, since all of our twenty-seven-year-old sleeping positions involve some sort of bodily contact.

There are oral appliances that can be inserted at bedtime. There is also an in-office medical procedure called somnoplasty, which, if I've got this right, uses radio frequency waves to melt the offending skin in the back of the throat, causing it to slough off naturally over the following weeks and months. More invasive surgeries and sprays are available, too, if none of the other things work.

To date I have refused to do the separate bed, separate room arrangement my grandparents utilized to solve this problem. But I am coming to agree more and more with Anne Shaw (at least in the louder night hours), who said, "Fond as we are of our loved ones, there comes at times during their absence an unexplained peace."

Emotionally Mature Men

He doesn't like to admit it, but David cries more now. I tease him about growing his "feminine" side—a normal and very real occurrence, given his (and every other middle-aged man's) receding male hormones.

This slight recalibration has put us closer than ever to the same emotional wavelength. Case in point: When our eldest son, Joshua, announced that God was leading him to leave his staff position at our church and take a new one at a large church up north, he might as well have said I'm off to Jupiter. We knew the position would be an honor for him (and for us), but the thought of whacking a mile-wide hole in our tight-knit ministry family was almost more than we could fathom. In the days following Josh's announcement, David and I could hardly be in the same room without inciting a stream of waterworks. And at night, it was not just me dripping tears on the pillow.

I'm still adjusting to it, but I think I like the comfort and closeness that comes from David's new ability to touch deeper emotions and let them flow out where I can see them. The word *commiserate* was probably coined at a time like this, when two parents were sharing a common grief over the moving out or away of one or more of their kids.

Another thing we do more now is talk about dying. When we were first married, we sometimes joked about what we would or would not do if one of us were to be suddenly taken out. But the reality of one of us dying seemed inconceivable back then. Now, every once in a while, David will mention that he occasionally stops to contemplate life without me as a way to prepare his heart for that day—which, in all stark truthfulness, is closer than we'd like to believe.

Whenever he gets to talking like that, I like to tease him and say, "Excuse me, sir. But I'm afraid the stats are in my favor. We both know it is highly likely that I will be the one left behind. And when that happens, I will finally be forced to learn how to balance a budget. Of course, the only budget I'll have to work with will come from your insurance money."

If you knew how horribly I handle finances (we're talking about a woman who runs down to the ATM machine and takes out twenty dollars just to find out how much money she has left in her account), you'd realize how frightening that runaway train is to my husband. And you'd understand why the mere hint of my living without him can get the man pretty choked up.

Watch for Flying Objects

Middle age, it seems, has a way of flushing out all kinds of emotions—including the nasty, unpleasant variety that wheedle their way to the forefront through various means. There's a reason people talk about the midlife crisis. As our age increases, we become like pots that have simmered on the stove too long. Sometimes the lid blows off.

In recent years the haphazard flow of my menstrual cycle has fueled some pretty hot arguments. One particularly strong one came not long after I started taking birth control pills to help readjust my hormones. Maybe the pills had nothing to do with it; maybe the circumstances were all that contributed to the situation heating up as much as it did. But later, after David and I both cooled off, the incident made me suspicious enough to back off the medication.

At this stage in life, many things come at us that have the power to sink, or at least rattle, even the best of marriages: erratic mood swings, irrational fears, career changes that create unstable finances, fluctuating libidos, physical illness, the stress of caring for aging parents, the stark silence left when the children move out and the parents find themselves without conversation filler for the first time in decades. Many of us experience several of these things at once. And if relational problems have been masked by years of busyness or distraction, the midlife passage, for some of us, becomes a deadly minefield.

The first half of 1995 was a season David and I would have

loved to skip. Because of an extremely painful and stressful time in our church, we were both going through a crisis at the same time. But the church trauma, it turned out, was only a catalyst for stirring up personal issues in us individually and as a couple that we just weren't ready to deal with—that is, until the heat on the stove got too hot to bear. What saved us from being fried beyond recognition was that we both agreed to break down and seek help. To this day we tell people that our decision to see a professional Christian counselor was one of the wisest calls we've ever made. The second half of 1995 became the dearest, most love-filled time of our marriage.

Since then David and I have moved even more to the center of our relationship from two very opposite points—he, the hyper, purpose-driven visionary; me, the lazy, creative contemplator. These days we are easy together, more patient, more tender. We share similar wavelengths now, similar visions. We see and appreciate one another's dreams. We want the other to be all he or she can be in this season, and we support and cheer for one another with gusto.

Save the Last Dance for Me

When it comes to the art of dancing, David and I wouldn't be worth watching, especially if you're talking the ballroom kind. But we have reached and mostly sustain a certain rhythm, an ease of sync that says, These two have covered some ground together—some of it hard and unsettling, most of it sweet and strong. They've weathered a bit, but well. See how each one anticipates the other with a certain fluid precision?

With practice, we can only get better. And that's good, because we still have more steps to learn.

👀 In the Chat Room

Leslie, 41: *"Talk about your emotions going off the Richter scale! I am a forty-one-year-old single mother of three, one of whom is graduating next month. A month after that, I am moving out of my first home and going to a new town with a new house, new husband, and new stepchildren. That's way too much going on at the same time while I'm still trying to hold down a full-time job! But overall I feel great and very ready. I am so thankful that God is giving me a second chance at marriage and has blessed me with the man of my dreams. I finally feel that feeling of being content."*

Martha, 49: *"My marriage is one of the most satisfying things in the aging process. It's very comforting to have that connection with the kids leaving home and my parents aging. I do have to remind myself to respond to my husband on the passion level, though, because that seems to remain very important to him—more so than to me. But he is very encouraging when I feel old and ugly. He still makes me feel desirable and attractive, and that helps me feel better about myself."*

Shirley, 40: *"Our intimate life is superb now compared to earlier years. We are totally comfortable with each other. I still want to look nice for my husband, and I still flirt with him."*

Mary Lou, 51: *"My faith is at a growing stage right now, and I wish I was sharing that growth with my husband."*

Lauren, 44: *"I find that I need a fifteen-minute nap at about four o'clock in the afternoon, and sometimes my husband and I snooze in front of the TV before bedtime—like his parents do!"*

Annette, 46: *"My husband and I seem to give each other more grace now. We're less reactive toward each other."*

Karen, 65: *"Making love with my husband isn't what it used to be, and it's not as often, but it still is sweet. It just isn't as important as it was. But we are more important to each other and grow dearer. I get concerned now and* then that we're reaching the age when we may not have each other one day. We cherish every moment together."

Susan, 49: "My eyesight is going. I have jiggly arms, and my legs look like a bad case of pudding. It amazes me that my husband still thinks I'm beautiful. At year twenty our marriage turned a corner—it was like everything clicked, and the last eight years have been the best ever. In fact, last Valentine's Day my husband had a CD made that was just about me and his love for me."

Praise the LORD, O my soul, and forget not all his benefits— who forgives all your sins and heals all your diseases, who redeems your life from the pit and crowns you with love and compassion, who satisfies your desires with good things so that your youth is renewed like the eagle's. (Ps. 103:2–5)

20

"Why are you so late?" asked the mother. "I had to help a girl who was in trouble," replied the daughter. "How did you help her?" "I sat dc vn and helped her cry." —Anonymous

A Little Whine Is Good for the Heart

The Bible says a lot of great things about keeping a positive attitude. We're encouraged to have a cheerful countenance, to rejoice, to be exceedingly glad, to sing, to clap, to dance. But sometimes, at certain significant crossings in life, the most profitable, productive, proactive thing a girl can do is have a good cry. And the Bible encourages that too.

Of course, the idea that it can be good to cry runs smack up against at least 84.5 percent of the training we received from our parents, teachers, and ninth-grade softball coaches. Not to mention many of the well-intentioned spiritual messages we've heard over the years. So what's a woman to do?

Good Grief

As you well know, the average female needs little coaxing to cry. Most of us have pretty much earned our emotional black belts by the age of thirteen. But the kind of crying I'm suggesting goes beyond random tears or occasional monthly weepiness. In fact, I'm convinced that, in order to move ahead and fully appreciate the multiplied joys of this season that some call "middle-escence," most of us will need to engage in a little "good grief."

What is good grief? Open the nearest Bible, dead center, and listen afresh to the copious cries of the King of Israel:

- "Give ear to my words, O LORD, consider my sighing." (Ps. 5:1)

- "Be merciful to me, LORD, for I am faint; O LORD, heal me, for my bones are in agony. My soul is in anguish. How long, O LORD, how long?…I am worn out from groaning; all night long I flood my bed with weeping and drench my couch with tears. My eyes grow weak." (Ps. 6:2–3, 6–7)

- "I am poured out like water, and all my bones are out of joint. My heart has turned to wax; it has melted away within me." (Ps. 22:14)

- "Turn to me and be gracious to me, for I am lonely and afflicted. The troubles of my heart have multiplied." (Ps. 25:16–17)

If these cries don't match, ailment for ailment, the lamentations of the average midlife woman, I don't know what does.

God's Take on Tears

But are these emotional displays really allowed? What does God think about them? I think it's safe to say that if such behavior were in any way offensive to God, somewhere in the book of 1 Chronicles we would read, "And...verily, verily, the ground opened up and swallowed King David, and he slept the sleep of his fathers forevermore."

But we see the exact opposite.

Against a backdrop of music and poetry, the Lord allows this crying king to wring out his heart like a dirty sponge. David makes no apologies. He never says, "Folks, I'm sorry. I really should get my act together." He admits that he's hot. Confused. That he's wearing a rut in the floor of his bed-chamber. We can imagine him shaking his fist or pounding the wall, eyes wet and bloodshot. His are the woes of a whipped warrior, a failed father, and a scorned shepherd. And if his cries teach us anything about this stretching, perplexing stage in our own lives, they teach us to go ahead and say where it hurts without shame.

Yes, you may be saying to yourself, *but King David's life was in danger, and his kingdom was in jeopardy. Compared to that, what are a little sagging skin, a few sleepless nights, and the kids heading out on their own?*

Most of us come from a long, long line of stiff-upper-lip, crying-will-get-you-nowhere sentiment. And while intended to make us strong, this kind of thinking may actually block us from experiencing the depth of emotional healing that can come from "constructive complaint."

There Is a Time to Mourn

Years ago, in a particularly dark time in my life, I spent a short season with a professional Christian counselor. During one session, as I was telling my story, I was surprised to see tears in the counselor's eyes.

"This is really sad, don't you think?" she said.

"Well, it's life," I said. "You get used to it." Then, thinking this was the proper, humble response, I added, "A lot of people have it much worse."

At that point the counselor said something that has marked the way I've tried to view all my troubles ever since.

"Sure, your stuff may not be as bad as someone else's," she said, "but we aren't talking about them. We're talking about you—your pain. You are allowed to feel sad. The things that happened were hurtful to you, and it's okay to say so. Don't pretend they had no effect. You will start feeling whole the day you let yourself grieve the losses."

Oh, I was good at letting *others* grieve. I'd say, "Take as long as you need to work through this. I totally understand." But when *I* was the one who was hurting, my self-talk said, "No use crying over spilled milk. Get with the program. Things could be worse. Why can't you look on the bright side?"

One of several reasons I had for writing this book was to help me process some of my own deep emotions about reaching middle life. Not all of my issues are devastating, but at times I have drifted into disillusionment over what feels like a series of robberies. Time has come and carted off my once naturally moisturized, wrinkle-free skin. It has shrunk my feminine hormones and healthy libido and reduced my fat burning power to T-minus zero and holding. It has brought me kicking and screaming (for the most part) to that sense-of-abandonment stage when parents must pass on and children must pass you up in favor of their own lives. At some point I know I'll need to stop and treat these flesh wounds.

What's All the Crying About?

But we're only talking about a few body and lifestyle changes, you may be thinking. Do they really warrant a pity party? After all, nobody's dying here.

Maybe no one is dying in the literal sense. But what do you call the dismantling of decades of intimate family life, or the throwing into reverse of relations with once-thriving parents? What about abrupt career changes, serious first-time health issues, or the realization that the person you used to see in the mirror is never coming back?

We like to quote Romans 8:28, and we certainly have the assurance that all things will work for good to those who love God and are called according to his purpose. But what should we do while we're waiting for that good to be worked out?

In her book *New Passages*, Gail Sheehy writes, "Psychologically something has to die before a new self can be born. We must come through something of a mourning phase to emerge and say, 'Okay, now I have a new life; there's a new part of me that is allowed to grow.'"[1] Yes, midlife should be all about forging ahead, blazing new trails. But in the process, many of us can expect to experience, to varying degrees, one or more authentic stages of grief, including feelings of denial, anger, isolation, and despair.

Am I saying we should allow ourselves to wallow in the swamp of self-absorption? Not at all. Nor am I advocating that we grieve a loss we truly don't feel or stay moody and distraught for prolonged periods. But we all process change at different rates and depths, and no two people will mourn the passing of the first stage of adulthood the same way. While one of my friends seems barely affected, another is convinced she will never recover. Maybe the best gift we can give our midlifing comrades (and ourselves) is permission to embrace this new season by first spending some time with sorrow.

We may need help. With so many different levels of change hitting us at once, the idea of slugging it out on our own can be immobilizing. Admitting this is not a sign of weakness or lack of spiritual maturity, any more than hiring a mechanic to adjust our brakes is a sign of ignorance. For some of us, getting the name of a good professional Christian counselor (most churches work in partnership with at least one) may just be the wisest, safest path we can take to help us sort things out.

Taking It to the Complaint Department

As we said earlier, King David is a great example of someone who knew how to express good grief. (Certain chapters of the Book of Psalms could almost be titled *A Manual for Midlife Mourners*.) Without qualifying his remarks, David dumped all of his troubles on God—and even at the height of his rawest emotions, God never scolded him or forbade him. Instead, the Father heard every groan. Then he planted them center stage, inside the most-read book of the most-read book in world history, giving us all a template for grieving our own transitions.

Do you, like David, need to express some good grief? If you're not sure, ask yourself the following questions:

- Do you lose sleep worrying, or vacillate between good and bad days when dealing with middle-life issues?

- Do you rehash events, repeatedly bringing up certain unchangeable situations, unable to move on?

- Is it possible that you are in denial (pretending you are fine) over an issue, hoping to avoid the pain of facing the truth? (You might confer with friends or family on this.)

- Do you spend part of your time fearful, angry, depressed, or dreading the future?

- Would others say you are not doing well with certain aspects of midlife?

- Do you consistently think and talk more about what you are losing than what you will be gaining?

If you answered yes to one or more of these, you probably have some issues you should take up with God. But how to begin? Follow David's example. He always took at least four steps whenever he visited the Royal Complaint Department:

1. He was specific about his complaints and feelings of grief.

2. He wept openly, giving voice to his pain.

3. He sang through his sorrow, applying music therapy to his soul.

4. He cried out to, counted on, and still praised God through the process.

At key valley moments in my own midlife passage, I'm finding that a little whine is good for my heart. If I didn't take time to express my frustration and sorrow, I think I would become emotionally crippled. I would poison the fruit that is mine for the picking in this new season God has for me.

To do this passage justice, each of us may need to carve out quality time for some good grief. I'm convinced that if it's done purposefully and honestly, in the presence of the Holy Spirit and perhaps among a few safe friends, our effort to say a deep, heartfelt good-bye to What Was might make saying hello to What's Next that much easier—and no doubt sweeter.

⊙ ⊙ In the Chat Room

Grace, 67: *"My biggest midlife challenge was a deep depression, but I didn't recognize it as such. I stopped going to church, didn't get out of bed. My husband just thought I had gotten lazy all of a sudden! I tell women to please try and get help. Talk to other women and to doctors. No one— including me—understood what was happening at the time."*

Susan, 49: *"My spiritual life helps me keep perspective and gives me vision. It grounds me for the tough times."*

Joann, 59: *"Both my parents are gone, and I've had to face a lot of issues related to my father. But God is bringing me healing and peace. I seem to have more hope for the future."*

Shirley, 40: *"Jesus is my best friend, and I talk to him about all the changes. Thank God he made me and knows what I'm going through! Since I'm just starting this journey, I plan to grab the hem of Jesus' garment and hold on for dear life."*

Lisa, 47: *"The fact that I have a relationship with Christ keeps me going. Because we walk by faith and trust and not by sight and feelings, I know he is in control. I count on the healing I find in him."*

There is a time...to weep and a time to laugh, a time to mourn and a time to dance. (Eccles. 3:1, 4)

A Time to Mourn

If you need help getting more definite closure on issues that are troubling you, try this prescription for good grief:

1. Buy a pack of 3x5 cards and pencil in an appointment with God.

2. When the appointment time arrives, take a card and write down one thing about this season that irritates, worries, or depresses you. Be as specific as possible. Take another card and write down another issue. Keep going until you run out of issues. (The number of cards you end up with isn't important.)

3. Divide all the cards into two stacks: Things I Can Do Something About, and Things I Have No Control Over.

4. On the backs of the Things I Can Do Something About cards, write down at least one practical way you will seek to work on resolving that issue.

5. On the back of the Things I Have No Control Over cards, write a Psalmlike prayer telling God exactly how you feel. (Use more than one card if you need to.)

6. Kneel or pace back and forth as you pray *aloud*, giving each matter over to God. Where you are angry, be angry. Where you are sad, fully grieve. Take your time. Don't hold back.

7. Repeat this as many times as it takes to come to a measure of peace on each issue. When you feel free, tear the card in half and throw it away.

8. If you continually struggle with a certain issue, don't assume it will go away on its own. Share it with a family member, ask several friends to pray with you, or see a pastor or counselor.

Midlife Survival Guide

When it comes to crossing the great Midlife Divide, it seems there aren't many previous experiences that prep us for this trek of ours—except maybe a go-round on a high-speed, hold-on-to-your-hat, hang-out-of-your-seat thrill ride.

Once a friend of mine dared herself to ride a certain roller coaster. It was one of those this-is-it, now-or-never-type dares. At a key adrenaline-stoked moment on the ride, this typically mature, demure woman, her eyes bolted shut, screamed to high heaven, "This was a stupid idea. Help me, Jeeeeesus! We're dead. I know we're all dead!"

But did she die? Not on your life. She got out of the car, redirected her bangs, grabbed a new ticket, and hopped right back on. And therein lies the parallel to our midlife adventure. It's one I'm definitely counting on: If we can just hang on till things level out, we're bound to see all the fun in it.

At your leisure, take a look at the list of midlife survival tips below. Nothing revolutionary; just a few little hints that may be helpful—especially on some of those thin-air, steep-incline days that are sure to be just around the corner:

1. *Keep moving.*

2. *Be often among safe, caring womenfolk. Watch yourself for growing isolation.*

3. *Upon waking say aloud, "Father, I know you are with me today. Your strong, loving Spirit is here right now. Come with me today, Father. Work through me. Teach me, and I will listen."*

4. *Listen to good music, morning and evening. Use it instead of food or television as a spirit booster.*

5. *Get out in the open air. Long walks do as much for the mind as for the body.*

6. *Fill your environments with all things live. Surround yourself with flowers, plants, people, nature, pets. (Live television does not count.)*

7. *Don't be afraid to write on your hand if you think you may forget something.*

8. *Buy clothes with 5 percent spandex.*

9. *As much as possible, only share meals with happy people.*

10. *Ask God's opinion first.*

11. *Be intelligent and sensible about your body. Do the research. Go the way of wisdom.*

12. *Do what gives you peace.*

13. *If you are really desperate, buy a cat.*

14. *Be often among children. Do things that cultivate childlike joy and playfulness.*

15. *Feel.*

16. *Give people as many chances as it takes for them to get it right. Jesus did.*

17. *Buy several good sun hats.*

18. *Drop lime slices in your water.*

19. *Increase your affection quotient. Give random hugs. Bear someone else's pain.*

20. *While washing your face, look in the mirror and say, "(Your*

name), you are beautiful, grace-filled, and priceless to God. You are the object of his affection. Yes, you are."

21. Buy new athletic shoes. You will walk faster and jump higher.

22. Find creative ways to be near water. Jesus did.

23. You already know about sunscreen.

24. Discover the elegance of three-quarter-length sleeves.

25. Stoke your private devotions. Recite meaningful scriptures. Pray aloud; talk like you would to a well-weathered friend. Write your prayers, or try using The Book of Common Prayer. Create your own worship songs. Open a hymnal and sing, or read the lyrics as poetry to God.

26. Wear only your best jewelry, but never all at once.

27. Set regular appointments to journal your life. Always write first about how you feel.

28. If things become unmanageable, talk with a professional Christian counselor. Shop around for the best fit. If your soul is infected, don't put off getting treatment.

29. Forgive on earth as you have been forgiven in heaven.

30. Replay funny, happy incidents with your family. Host a "Remember When" night.

31. Find a teenage girl who reminds you of you, and mentor her.

32. Participate in a life-giving church—one that celebrates, teaches, and loves Jesus Christ and people like you.

33. Invest your resources in things that will last.

34. Choose a signature color. Wear it often. Buy small, personal items in this color. Use it to paint a wall or even your front door.

35. At the start of each month, make yourself finish this sentence: "One thing I would really like to do this month is _____."

36. Tell your troubles to Jesus. Dump the whole truck in his lap. He can take it.

37. Embrace the wow of Now. Open up. Welcome its presence. See what's there. Rejoice in all its fresh, sweet, juicy possibilities.

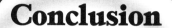

Conclusion

Continuity gives us roots.
Change gives us branches.
—Pauline R. Kezer

My Prayer for
Your Passage

A lot of women don't care much for change. You really can't blame them. Change can be so rude. It never says, "Oh dear, sorry for the inconvenience. This will only take a second." Just when we've finally arrived somewhere, change has the nerve to reach down, release the safety brake, and make us go frantic— like a mom with a runaway stroller.

From a young age, change for me was rarely about adventure, discovery, or fresh beginnings. It seemed my changes were always barging in, like a riot of drunken sailors who never paid for damages. I was a skittish child living in a state of "brace," eyes sharply peeled for the next jarring pothole in the road.

Controlling my surroundings and taking the long way around new things were my best coping tools, even into adulthood. I wanted familiar people or places or circumstances (or even now, a familiar body in the mirror) to keep me grounded. In those days I had not yet heard that the God Who Never Changes was in the neighborhood. I didn't know that—after all was said and done—he would turn out to be the only true anchor in the vast, unpredictable sea that is this life.

But now I do know. And I've arrived at the place where to live full-out, I must live and breathe change. The question is, how am I going to handle it?

Dressing for Success

There is still so much about this transition that I'm trying to bring into focus. I am closer than ever to—yet still a bit east of—Mount Menopause, and to be honest, I'm not quite sure how I will act when I finally get there. I had gotten fairly attached to my former skin, and now I feel like a naked she-snake coiled on a rock, waiting for new scales to grow.

What I do know is this: All will not be foreign in this new world. It's like each new fashion season. Styles change, and sometimes we cringe when the tops come out sleeveless or the hemlines rise near flood level. But no matter our age, each season still manages to bring color and fabrics and several great styles that seem to suit us just fine.

And just as clothing trends often mimic earlier times, so it is with the changing wardrobe of our lives at this halfway point. Even here we see things familiar. Many tried-and-true options still work for us. There are anchor points, too, especially if we have asked the Rock of Ages to be the buyer and keeper of our closet.

The Incredible Journey

You and I are about to embark on the journey of a lifetime. And that means we've got some packing to do.

The experts say it's smart to pack light, so we'll need to decide what to keep and what to toss because they'd only slow us down. We'll need to get in shape, pick travel buddies, sharpen old skills, learn some new ones, test our gear, shop for rations, study our map, say some good-byes—and then start on down the road.

From the girls up ahead comes this postcard back to us: "All is well. Come soon! You won't believe the view."

So as you go on in your own God-marked way, I speak this last prayer over you:

Lord,
Help this special sister to sleep like a child through
the earthquakes.
Help her waltz on the shifting sand and stay loose
through the rugged detours—even those she must take in the
dark.
May she walk to the lead of your still, small voice.
Let her smile at the rising sun,
And may she steer in the night by those stars you have
hung just for her.

Happy hiking, dear sister. Last one to the top is a rotten egg.

The path of the righteous is like the first gleam of dawn, shining ever brighter till the full light of day. (Prov. 4:18)

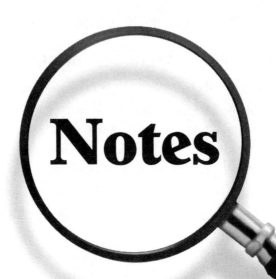

Chapter 2: Has Anyone Seen My Hormones?

1. Gail Sheehy, *New Passages: Mapping Your Life Across Time* (New York: Ballantine Books, 1995), 207.

2. Ibid., 206–207.

Chapter 3: Wombs to Go

1. Letty Cottin Pogrebin, *Getting Over Getting Older* (New York: Berkley Books, 1996), 198.

Chapter 5: Everybody's Doing the Birthday Bash

1. Carolyn Warner, *Treasury of Women's Quotations* (Englewood Cliffs, N. J.: Prentice Hall, 1992), 18.

Chapter 7: Huffin' with the Health-Club Hotties

1. Christiane Northrup, *The Wisdom of Menopause* (New York: Bantam Books, 2001), 195.

2. Ibid., 194–95.

Chapter 17: Midlife Goes to the Dogs

1. "The State of the American Pet: A Study Among Pet Owners" [online]. Healthy Pets 21 Consortium, Purina Pet Institute, October 2000 [cited 6 December, 2002]. Portable Document Format. Available from: http://www.purina.com/images?articles/pdf/TheStateofthe.pdf

Chapter 20: A Little Whine Is Good for the Heart

1. Sheehy, *New Passages: Mapping Your Life*, 145.